Modification and Preservation of Existing Dental Restorations

Donald W. Fisher, D.D.S.
Clinical Professor and Chairman
Fixed Prosthodontics
University of California at Los Angeles School of Dentistry

William W. Morgan, D.D.S.
Lecturer, Fixed Prosthodontics
University of California at Los Angeles School of Dentistry
and Private Practice
Woodland Hills, California

Quintessence Publishing Co., Inc. 1987
Chicago, Berlin, London, São Paulo, Hong Kong, and Tokyo

Library of Congress Cataloging-in-Publication Data

Fisher, Donald W., 1936–
  Modification and preservation of existing dental
restorations.

  Includes bibliographies and index.
  1. Dentistry, Operative. 2. Prosthodontics.
I. Morgan, William W. (William Wilson), 1945–
II. Title. [DNLM: 1. Dental Restoration, Permanent—
methods. WU 300 F533m]
RK501.F53 1987   617.6′9   86-9427
ISBN 0-86715-131-5

Lithography: Industrie- und Presseklischee, Berlin, and Sun Art Printing Co., Osaka
Composition: Midwest Technical Publications, Inc., St. Louis, MO
Printing and binding: Worzalla Publishing Company, Stevens Point, WI
Printed in U. S. A.

Dedicated To Gloria Fisher and
Karen Morgan

For their support, understanding, and encourage-
ment, without which this book would not have been
possible

The professional man has no right to be other than a continuous student.

G.V. Black

Contents

Contents

Foreword

Restorative dentistry can be very complex, and the more complicated it becomes, the greater the chance that something may go wrong. Complex dental treatment is also very expensive, and remakes are costly, whether they are the responsibility of the patient or of the dentist. The patient and dentist alike benefit if the remake of an existing restoration can be *reasonably* avoided. Although we all modify and preserve restorations in our practices, this book gives guidelines and techniques for doing this while maintaining a high level of quality.

This is not a quick-fix manual for doing patchwork dentistry. It is a well-thought-out approach to diagnosing common restorative failures and distinguishing those that are amenable to modification from those that require remakes. Step-by-step instructions are given for producing restorations of equal or higher quality than they were originally, while adhering to the basic tenets of quality restorative dental care.

This is a book for the clinical dentist. It is authored by two especially well-qualified dentists who have devoted their careers to both practicing and teaching dentistry. Their experience in practice provides them with a first-hand knowledge of the problems faced by clinicians, while their experience in teaching gives them an excellent background in analyzing those problems and providing solutions in ways which are easy to comprehend.

Experienced practitioners and novices alike will find this book well worth reading. It gives alternate ways of correcting problems encountered in every dental practice, such as how to preserve a restoration made last year, or how to preserve one 20 years old, possibly made with materials no longer in manufacture, or by techniques no longer used.

Why hasn't this book been written before? To ask this question is like observing the grace with which an Olympic skater glides across the ice saying, "That looks easy." But apparent ease and simplicity stem from the thousands of hours of practice spent developing the skills displayed.

Herbert T. Shillingburg, Jr.

Preface

In the past 70 years, the dental profession has undergone so many major changes that the practice of dentistry only vaguely resembles what it was prior to that time. Exceptionally dramatic strides have been made in the ability of the dental practitioner to save teeth and restore them to proper function. Many procedures that were unheard of in the recent past are done routinely now.

The development in 1907 of techniques that allowed dentists to use cast gold as an effective and reliable restorative material was a major breakthrough in modern dentistry. Later, the introduction of, and ongoing improvements in, modern impression materials made it possible to obtain a very accurate cast of a prepared tooth and to thereby increase the accuracy and fit of its dental casting.

Much progress has also been made in preventive dentistry. The use of fluoride in many forms has drastically reduced the incidence of dental caries and the ensuing loss of teeth. In addition, knowledge about the cause, prevention, and treatment of periodontal disease has enabled patients to retain teeth that would have been lost a generation or two ago.

Another factor responsible for saving more teeth has been the development and acceptance of endodontic therapy. Since the early 1950s, when safe and reliable endodontic techniques were being perfected, many teeth that previously would have been extracted have been retained and restored. Patient acceptance of endodontic therapy has now increased to the point where it is performed routinely in many offices.

Other developments, such as high-speed rotary instrumentation, porcelain-fused-to-metal restorations, and improvements in direct-filling materials, have greatly improved the quality of dental care. In addition, the increased availability and use of third-party providers in recent years has made quality dental care affordable to more people. In previous years many teeth would simply have been extracted rather than restored, due to patients' financial considerations.

In dentistry, there is usually a lag time between the development of a new technique and its acceptance by the profession. Once accepted, there is often another time lapse before dentists appreciate and understand the finer principles of the new technique. In addition, ongoing research is always producing improvements in techniques and materials. These factors can result in restorations that are not as well placed as subsequent ones will be. Fortunately, such early examples of a new technique can sometimes be modified and preserved.

As a result of these previously mentioned developments, an increased number of dental restorations have been placed, some of which have developed defects after a reasonable period of time. Today it is usually possible to replace a previous restoration and save the tooth; this is often the best treatment because many methods of "fixing" defective restorations are not in a patient's best interest.

Sometimes, however, it may be preferable to retain an existing restoration by modifying it. The advantages of saving an existing restoration may be psychological, economic, esthetic, or functional. Several methods for modifying existing restorations will be presented in this book. *It is strongly emphasized that the techniques advocated here are aimed at producing high-quality restorations. A modified restoration must be as good as or better than it was when originally placed.* The techniques presented are not quick fixes, but are very exacting and, in some cases, time-consuming procedures. In some situations the added effort is not only justified, it is the best treatment for the patient.

Many dental practitioners have been faced with decreased patient loads. Some in the profession might ask: Why not simply replace a defective restoration instead of going to the trouble to modify it, especially when modification is generally less lucrative financially? The answer lies in the dentist's ethical obligation to provide the care that is in the best interest of the patient. If the dentist can avoid unnecessary treatment by modifying an existing restoration—and produce high-quality results—then the patient should be offered that alternative.

This book puts forth specific clinical situations and various alternatives for treatment. The procedures included will give predictable results when followed correctly. But practitioners must evaluate all possible alternatives, including those not given here in detail, by applying sound principles of restorative dentistry.

Techniques presented here are intended to be performed by general dentists and prosthodontists—those practitioners normally doing restorative dentistry. Procedures to be performed by other specialists and dental laboratory technicians are not included in this text, except in passing reference, since they are adequately covered in other sources. Many dental technicians will be familiar with the applicable laboratory procedures, but clinicians should verify that their technicians can accomplish the appropriate steps before they attempt these procedures.

Also excluded from this book are questionable techniques that do not conform to basic principles of restorative dentistry, methods that would likely result in poor restorations, unusual or relatively complicated procedures such as precision attachments and implants, and relatively new techniques such as acid-etched bridges.

Each chapter and section is intended to stand alone. The illustrations and clinical photographs serve as aids for following the various techniques, but are not intended to provide a full understanding of the procedures if studied apart from the accompanying text.

The chapter on adjunct techniques describes various procedures that have multiple applications. Some of these procedures are new and may not have been taught in dental schools until very recently. Many of these techniques are helpful in routine restorative procedures, and can be incorporated into general practice.

As patients continue to have more teeth restored and thereby retained, the dentist will be faced with an increased number of patients with existing restorations that are failing. Instead of automatically replacing them, the dentist should be aware of other alternatives and the criteria that must be satisfied in order to modify and preserve them. This text is intended to expand the dentist's range of treatment alternatives so that patients can be offered the widest possible range of treatment choices.

Acknowledgments

We gratefully acknowledge the assistance of Irene Petravicius of the UCLA Dental Illustration Department for her excellent original drawings throughout this work. Her creativity and efficiency were great assets to us. We also thank Richard Friske, Catherine Siegel, and B. J. Coburn of the UCLA Dental Photography Department for their assistance in producing the photographs.

While much of the knowledge required to produce a work of this type must come from research papers and other printed materials, interpretation of this material is greatly aided by one's association with former teachers as well as colleagues, past and present. Among these is Dr. Robert Dewhirst, a clinician with few peers, whose constant search for better modes of treatment and insistence on the highest quality have been guiding forces in our thinking.

Another is Dr. Herbert T. Shillingburg, Jr., a truly excellent teacher, whose philosophies and knowledge have been an inspiration for many years to us and to dentists all over the world. Another fine teacher is Dr. Robert Wolcott, who has been an example to students and colleagues with his impeccable standards of patient care, as well as a recognized leader in the field of dental education. Dr. Robert Vig epitomizes the dentist who places patient needs at the forefront in his treatment choices. Not the least of these is Dr. W. E. Fisher, a practicing dentist for 50 years, who gave living meaning to the idea of putting the patient's needs above all other concerns. To these men, and others like them, we owe an inestimable debt of gratitude for providing us with a foundation of principles on which to base the various thoughts put forth in this book.

Chapter 1

General Principles

Changes in the practice of dentistry

During the 20th century, many professions and vocations have either been created or have dramatically evolved due to changing technology. The dental profession has undergone major changes, from one in which the dentist-barber removed painful teeth, to a highly skilled discipline aimed at preserving complete oral health. Many factors have played roles in this evolution, including: knowledge and skills in preventive dentistry; new restorative techniques; improved materials; specialization training, including expanded duties of dental personnel; and an overall desire on the part of the public for high-quality, affordable dental care concurrent with the increase in ability to afford better care.

Prevention

Knowledge of the causes of periodontal disease and its prevention, as well as treatment advances, have had a major impact on the practice of dentistry. Many teeth are now being saved for a much longer time, which leads to a decreased need for full denture prosthodontics, but an increased need for fixed prosthodontics.

The function of dental plaque in the development of dental disease has been clearly demonstrated, and dentists no longer recommend that periodic scaling and polishing is sufficient for

saving teeth. Instead, the patient is encouraged to participate in maintaining good oral health. In many cases the patient's role is more critical than that of the dentist, since the dentist cannot compensate for what the patient will not do.

At the onset of periodontal disease, oral hygiene is even more critical. Advances in treatment of periodontal defects can stop the progression of the disease and allow patients to maintain their natural dentition. Periodontal surgery, which reduces or eliminates deep pockets, gives access to areas which the patient was previously unable to clean, and thereby provides an opportunity to retain teeth which would have been lost in an earlier generation.

The increased use of fluoride in all forms, including fluoridated water, fluoridated toothpaste, as well as topical applications of fluoride in the dental office, has significantly reduced dental caries. Studies have shown that up to 65% of caries can be prevented by proper use of fluoride.[1] While fluoride prevents smooth surface lesions and eventually reduces the need for future cast restorations, root caries and recurrent caries continue to provide challenges for dentists, particularly as related to existing restorations.[2]

Endodontic therapy is also significant. The development of safe and reliable methods of this therapy have given highly predictable and successful results. Today, most dentists either do endodontics themselves, or refer such patients to an endodontist when this treatment is indicated.

While most patients still approach root canal treatment with a little trepidation, such treatment is perceived as an accepted alternative to extraction. As a result, there are numerous teeth still retained which otherwise would need to be removed. Some teeth are not restorable except for the additional retention afforded by the use of the endodontically treated canal.

Restorative techniques

A second major development which has had an impact on dentistry is in the area of new restorative techniques. Once dentists were able to cast gold precisely and predictably, a whole new area of restorative dentistry opened. Cast gold crowns can be used to restore teeth with a comparatively high degree of accuracy and ease. Previously, the tooth was either extracted, restored with a "filling" of some sort, or a crown was adapted to it by swedging or burnishing, which was a very laborious and inaccurate process. When these restorations failed, frequently the only alternative was extraction. When a modern restoration fails, the dentist can often either modify or replace it and still retain the tooth most of the time.

Another significant restorative technique is the process of baking porcelain to metal. This has allowed dentists to create a crown or a fixed bridge which is more esthetic and durable than acrylic or other types of porcelain facings.

When porcelain-fused-to-metal restorations were introduced, high-speed rotary instrumentation was also becoming more popular. It became possible to cut preparations on teeth in only a fraction of the time previously required. With a water spray to cool the tooth, restorative procedures could be accomplished with greater patient comfort and less trauma to the pulp of the tooth. These changes have led to increased patient acceptance of necessary treatment.

Improvements in materials

Since the introduction of dental castings, there have been tremendous improvements in dental materials. Instead of direct waxups in the mouth, a very difficult and questionably accurate procedure, dentists can now choose among several highly accurate impression materials including reversible hydrocolloid, polysulfide rubber base, silicones, and the newer polyvinylsiloxanes and polyethers.

There have also been changes in the casting alloys. Owing to the high cost of gold, several alternative alloys have been developed. Although using them is more difficult than using gold, they can produce excellent results within their limitations. In addition to being less expensive, some of the semiprecious and nonprecious alloys in porcelain fused to metal restorations actually have some qualities superior to those of alloys with a high gold content.[3]

Filling materials have also changed. With the introduction of the visible light cured composites, there are materials which are more esthetic, stronger, and more color-stable than previously used silicates, acrylics, and conventional composites. These materials will also take a reasonably good finish. With the acid etch technique, they are very stable in terms of marginal seal.[4]

Amalgam has also changed. High copper dispersion phase alloys have been shown to retain high marginal integrity several years after proper placement.[5] However, the best available material will not make up for poor technique. It is still necessary to prevent moisture contamination preferably by using the rubber dam, which also improves working conditions.

Advanced training

Highly trained dental personnel can enable today's dentists to diagnose and treat more patients in a shorter time. Many procedures previously done by the dentist can now be delegated to auxiliary personnel.

Dental hygienists, with their two-year specialized training program, are a real asset in today's dental office. They can spend time the dentist cannot afford to spend thoroughly scaling and polishing teeth, as well as teaching and motivating patients in proper oral hygiene.

Recent years have also seen an increase in specialty training and other postgraduate dental training. The public is receiving higher-quality dental care because of such specialization and the general dentist who performs treatment that could be referred to a specialist is obligated to provide the same level of care offered by the specialist. Thus a dentist must keep abreast of the latest developments and trends in whatever areas he or she chooses to practice.

In order to provide the best patient care, it is not enough for dentists to attend four years of dental school and then use the same methods and techniques indefinitely. Instead dentists are obligated to participate in continuing education programs to stay current. Dental meetings, up-to-date textbooks, articles in reputable journals, and courses offered through dental schools or other agencies can all help the modern dentist stay abreast of new developments.

Patient attitude changes

Patients are becoming more aware that extractions are frequently unnecessary, and their desire for higher quality care is increasing. They more often choose endodontic treatment and a crown rather than extraction for the symptomatic, broken-down tooth.

In addition to patients' desires for a higher caliber of dental care, there is the ability for them to afford this higher quality treatment. This has resulted from a general economic upswing as well as an ever-increasing portion of the population that has dental insurance or other third-party payment plans, conditions that have somewhat compensated for the decreased incidence of dental caries.

Evaluating the quality of existing restorations

An evaluation of existing restorations will lead to one of three possible courses:

1. The first is to leave the restoration untreated. This choice should be made when there are no defects whatsoever or when any defects are so inconsequential that to neglect them would not lead to any further breakdown of the healthy tooth or surrounding tissue. Although this is the most common choice by far, it must not be arrived at by default. Instead, a careful examination is necessary to rule out any defects.

2. The second course is to replace the restoration. This choice will result from a defect or combination of defects that if neglected would lead to further breakdown of the tooth or surrounding tissues. The existing restoration is not amenable to modification.

3. The third alternative is to modify the existing restoration in order to preserve it. This choice is *sometimes* available when a defect requiring treatment is discovered. This has been a relatively uncommon course, though it is increasingly becoming a treatment of choice.

In each technique presented, certain criteria must be met. Otherwise, the restoration must be remade. It is important to recognize that the standards applied to an existing restoration are different from those applied to one being placed initially. Defects which would make a new restoration unacceptable do not necessarily require remaking an existing restoration. Factors such as length of time a restoration has been in place with a minor defect (a defect that has not produced untoward results such as caries or periodontal disease), age and medical history of the patient, and severity of the defect need to be considered before deciding to remake the restoration.

However, whenever an existing restoration is modified and therefore preserved, *the resulting restoration should be as good if not better than when it was originally placed*. The criteria applied here are the same that the dentist should apply when making new restorations. For example, a patient presented with acrylic-faced crowns that had failing margins, worn facings that no longer fit the existing partial denture, and poor tissue response (Fig. 1-1a). The patient

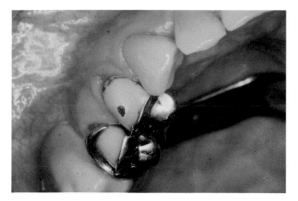

Fig. 1-1a Defective acrylic-faced crowns under partial denture.

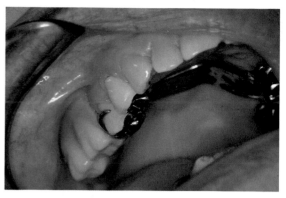

Fig. 1-1b New porcelain-fused-to-metal crowns under the same partial denture.

was satisfied with the partial denture, which was well-made and properly functioning. By following the outlined procedure in the chapter on crowns under removable partial dentures, two porcelain-fused-to-metal crowns were fabricated with porcelain instead of acrylic for clasp retention, had well-fitting margins, and resulted in improved esthetics and tissue response (Fig. 1-1b).

Several clinical factors must be evaluated when examining any restoration. A satisfactory restoration must meet the acceptable criteria in the following areas: function, contour, esthetics, margins, occlusion, and pulpal, periapical, and periodontal health.

Function

The first question to ask when evaluating existing restorations is: Does the restoration function as intended? For example, if the restoration is a fixed bridge or removable partial denture replacing several posterior teeth, the patient should be able to chew painlessly, efficiently, and without damaging the teeth or surrounding tissues (Figs. 1-2a and b). If the restoration is malfunctioning, or if the patient is dissatisfied, further examination is necessary to determine the cause. If the cause cannot be determined, it is possible that a replacement will also be unsat-

isfactory. This is particularly true for removable partial dentures. Patient satisfaction is harder to achieve in this area, even when the prosthesis is technically correct.

However, when a patient is happy with a removable partial or full denture which has a correctable defect, preserving the appliance by correction or modification should be seriously considered. Attaining the same level of patient satisfaction with a new appliance may be difficult. The dentist must use his or her professional judgment in deciding when an existing appliance is no longer acceptable.

Contours

When evaluating contours of an existing restoration, observe the color, form, and surface texture of the surrounding gingival tissue. An overcontoured crown can cause inflamed and swollen gingiva that will lead to more serious periodontal involvement (Fig. 1-3). However, gingival inflammation which results from poor oral hygiene usually should not require a new restoration unless the crown makes good oral hygiene difficult or impossible.

A poor contour is shown in Figure 1-4a. One can see the following defects in the maxillary right central incisor: (1) The incisal length is too

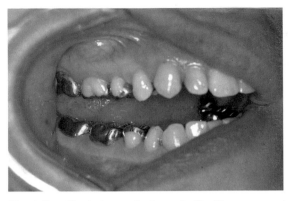

Fig. 1-2a Posterior occlusion rebuilt with crowns.

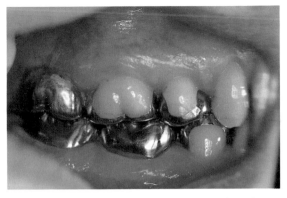

Fig. 1-2b Posterior crowns in proper functional relationship.

great and corners are too nearly square; (2) the mesial and distal facial line angles are too far apart, making the tooth appear too wide; and (3) the gingival contour is not conducive to good tissue health.

This situation was corrected with a new restoration (Fig. 1-4b). Note the following improvements: (1) the incisal length and shape are more harmonious with the contralateral tooth; (2) the width of the facial surface is more like the contralateral tooth; and (3) the gingival tissue is healthy.

In addition to observing the gingival appearance, the periodontal tissues must be carefully

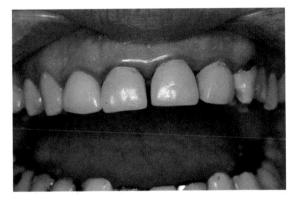

Fig. 1-3 Poor contour resulting in unfavorable gingival response.

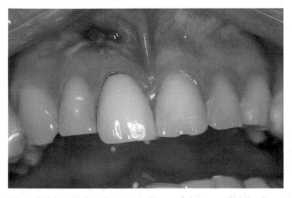

Fig. 1-4a Defective maxillary right central incisor crown.

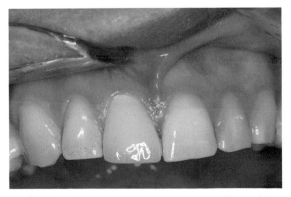

Fig. 1-4b Replacement crown for maxillary right central incisor with defects corrected.

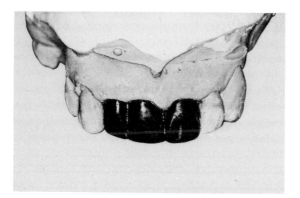

Fig. 1-5 Diagnostic waxup for maxillary anterior crowns.

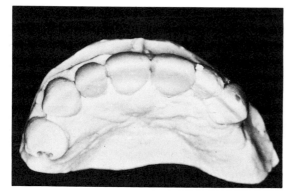

Fig. 1-6a Temporary crowns made from diagnostic waxup.

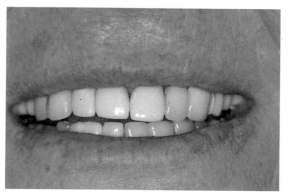

Fig. 1-6b Temporary crowns in patient.

examined with the periodontal probe, and any pockets noted and measured. Another essential aid in this part of the examination is a set of full-mouth radiographs. Both the development of pockets and the increase in pocket depth may be caused by poorly contoured restoration.

Overcontoured crowns often result from inadequate axial reduction of the tooth by the dentist, and the only solution is to make a new crown after correcting the preparation. However, overcontoured crowns can also result from laboratory error, which would necessitate a new crown.

Poor contours or tooth positions can cause chronic cheek or tongue-biting. This can happen when maxillary and mandibular posterior teeth have inadequate facial or lingual overlap. Simple recontouring of the involved surfaces of one or the other arches will sometimes alleviate

this, but at other times repositioning the tooth orthodontically or remaking the restoration is needed.

Contour and tooth position are critical factors in the anterior area, and improper restorations can cause phonetic difficulty. For example, a change in contour or tooth position can affect a musician's ability to produce certain sounds from a brass or woodwind instrument.

Whenever anterior crown and bridge treatment is planned, a diagnostic waxup is strongly recommended (Fig. 1-5). From this waxup temporary restorations are made and proper contours and tooth position can be determined (Figs. 1-6a and b). The temporary restorations can be modified by adjusting or adding new acrylic until the proper form is achieved. Then the final restorations can be made using either the diagnostic waxup, or a model of the tempo-

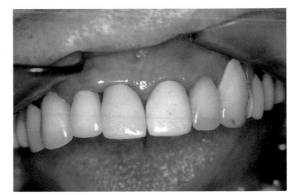

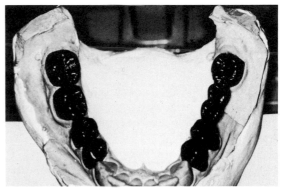

Fig. 1-7 Same patient with permanent crowns on right central and lateral incisors and temporary crown on left central incisor.

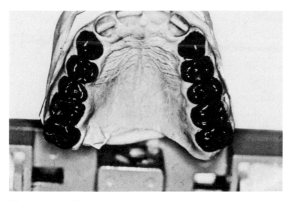

Fig. 1-8a Maxillary view of posterior diagnostic waxup.

Fig. 1-8b Mandibular view of posterior diagnostic waxup.

raries if they have been modified, as a guide to proper contour and tooth position. If this procedure for making temporaries is followed by both the dentist and the technician, the temporary and final restorations will be interchangeable (Fig. 1-7). This procedure is particularly important when treating musicians or individuals who do extensive public speaking. It is much easier to discover functional problems when the patient is still wearing temporaries which can easily be modified, rather than making such discoveries after the final restorations are cemented when the only alternative is to remake them. In this case, unless a diagnostic waxup is used, even the remake may not eliminate the problem.

When extensive posterior cast restorations are planned, a diagnostic waxup is invaluable. Proper contours and occlusal relationships can

be determined in advance, and the temporary restorations can maintain these relationships (Figs. 1-8a and b).

Esthetics

Patients are becoming increasingly concerned with the effect of their dentition on their appearance. Ideally, restorations in highly visible areas maintain proper function and are virtually undetectable (Fig. 1-9). However, an esthetically poor restoration can be obvious to even the casual observer (Fig. 1-10). Usually, only slight esthetic modifications can be made to existing restorations. A major discrepancy in shade, shape, or size is unattractive and so usually requires replacement.

An existing restoration, however, may be very

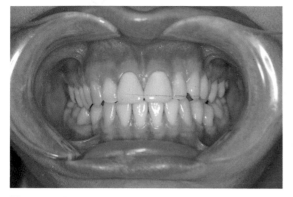

Fig. 1-9 Three maxillary anterior porcelain-fused-to-metal crowns.

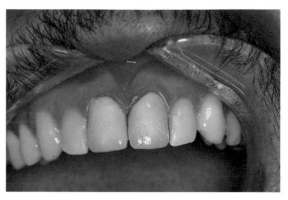

Fig. 1-10 Unesthetic maxillary central incisor crowns.

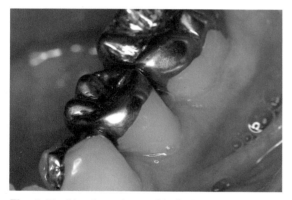

Fig. 1-11 Nearly undetectable facial margins.

difficult to match, particularly with regard to shade. The multiple and often conflicting problems of hue, value, and translucency are involved. When a previous restoration has been successful in a difficult esthetic situation, there is an incentive to correct a minor defect if possible, and avoid a remake.

Margins

One of the most critical determinants of a successful dental restoration is the marginal relationship. The standard for every dentist is for the crown to perfectly fit the tooth. The tooth/crown interface should not be easily detected (Fig. 1-11). Usually, the accuracy of the fit is determined by probing for defects with an explorer; if

none are discovered the fit is assumed to be satisfactory.

However, there can be significant discrepancies that go undetected when checking only with an explorer, because their design and sharpness vary (Fig. 1-12). An older explorer which has been dulled with use will miss an even greater defect than a new sharp one will (Fig. 1-13). For the dentist to simply check the margin with an explorer can lead to overconfidence, and therefore the margins should be checked for closeness of fit by more precise methods wherever possible. A much smaller opening between tooth and crown can be better detected visually, preferably with magnification, than can be felt with an explorer. All supragingival margins should be checked this way (Fig. 1-14). Also, interproximal marginal defects can sometimes be detected on bitewing radiographs (Fig. 1-15), though this method should not be used exclusively (Fig. 1-16).

Any of these methods can be used to check the fit of a crown prior to cementation. They are the only options for examining the marginal fit of an already cemented crown. However, the best time to ascertain whether crowns fit well is long before cementation.

When the tooth is prepared, the dentist should carefully create definite, reproducible finish lines. There is also no substitute for an accurate impression that reproduces all marginal areas. The stereomicroscope can be used

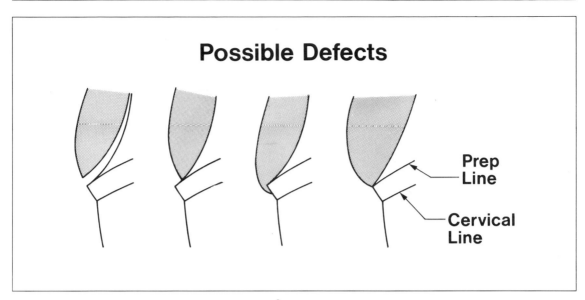

Fig. 1-12 Defects at the crown-to-tooth junction that might be located by the explorer.

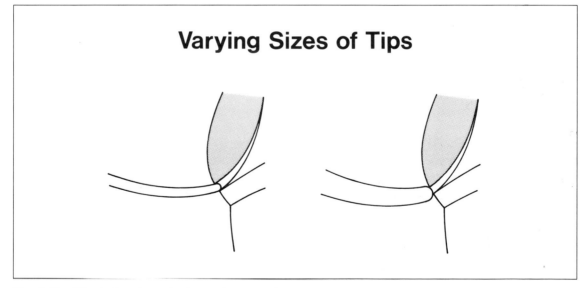

Fig. 1-13 Effect of explorer tip size on location of openings at margins.

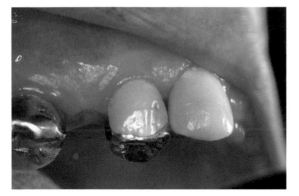

Fig. 1-14 Open margin on casting.

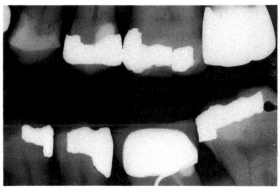

Fig. 1-15 Radiograph showing open margin on distal portion of mandibular first molar.

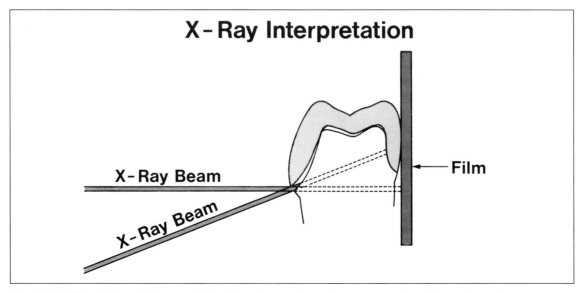

Fig. 1-16 Effect of angulation on ability to locate openings at crown margins using radiographs.

to determine whether all finish lines are reproduced, and that they are accurately trimmed on the die. The stereomicroscope also allows the technician to be more precise during both waxing and fitting the crown to the die. Various marking media, such as a machinist's marking dye or reline washes are highly functional at the clinical try-in step. Not only are open margins visible with this technique, but the magnitude and geometric form of the defect also can be observed and evaluated (Figs. 1-17a to c). For

more information regarding these techniques, refer to the section on the stereomicroscope in chapter 9.

When an open margin is discovered, the crown should almost always be replaced. When the defect is limited to a small portion of the marginal area and represents a specific, isolated, and identifiable opening rather than being the result of a poorly fitting crown, it may be possible to correct the defect. Factors such as duration in the mouth, its relationship to other

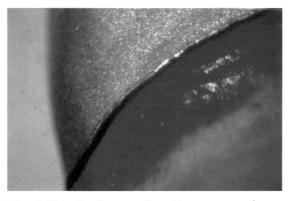

Fig. 1-17a Casting on die with open margin as viewed under the stereomicroscope.

restorative dentistry, esthetics, overall caries rate, and the age and health of the patient may enter into this decision. Good clinical judgment is necessary and there are no absolute answers which will apply in every case. As in any other area of dentistry, the primary consideration should be what is best for the patient.

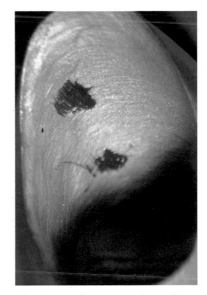

Fig. 1-17b Internal aspect of casting showing marks indicating areas of interference with seating.

Occlusion

Occlusion is one of the most controversial and least appreciated areas of dentistry. Opinions regarding proper occlusal schemes are wide-ranging, and much has been written on the subject. Proper occlusion allows for normal function without leading to any pathology in any area related to the tooth support, temporomandibular joints, or related tissues. Wear facets on occlusal surfaces, widened periodontal ligament space, or mobility of the teeth can be caused by malocclusion. Degeneration of or symptoms in the temporomandibular joints may indicate occlusal problems and must be investigated by proper patient history and thorough oral examination.

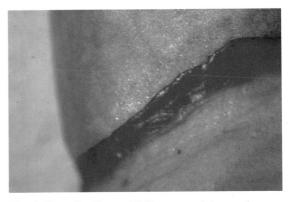

Fig. 1-17c Casting exhibiting complete seating as viewed under the stereomicroscope after adjustment to remove interferences.

When treating occlusal problems prior to restorative procedures, the occlusion needs to be stabilized and acute symptoms must be under control. Diagnostic casts of these patients should be mounted in retruded, that is, terminal hinge position by using proper facebow-mounting techniques, interocclusal recordings, and

protrusive records. Where indicated, a pantographic tracing should be made.

These relationships also need to be proven with a second set of occlusal records. By doing this, an accurate evaluation of the patient occlusion can be made and proper treatment planning accomplished. Whenever significant occlusal changes are considered, such as multiple fixed prosthodontic restorations, the same procedure should be followed. In addition to prop-

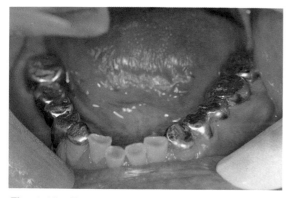

Fig. 1-18 Extreme wear on occlusal surfaces of crowns.

erly mounted diagnostic casts, occlusal indicating wax and marking tape or ribbon can help locate any occlusal interferences which may cause pathological changes.

It may be possible to modify existing restorations with occlusion problems. If this is impossible, the defective restoration must be replaced. Crowns with severe wear may not be preservable, and perforations in these situations would necessitate replacement (Fig. 1-18). Small facets, however, can be eliminated and in some cases a perforation can be restored when the surrounding metal has adequate thickness.

When a crown with an occlusal problem has another correctable deficiency, the occlusal problem should usually be treated and eliminated first unless the other defect is causing an acute problem that demands immediate treatment. The corrected occlusion can be evaluated, and if deemed satisfactory in relation to symptomatology, the other defect can be addressed. If occlusal stability cannot be accomplished with the existing restoration it should be replaced.

Pulpal, periapical, and periodontal considerations

Before attempting to make any of the corrections described in the text, it is essential to be as

nearly certain as possible that periapical and pulpal disease is absent in the area to be affected by the treatment. While it is impossible to be absolutely certain that the pulp is healthy, its status should still be determined as accurately as possible. A conscientious dentist will not do a crown without a thorough clinical and radiographic examination. When deciding to correct or modify an existing crown, it is equally important to use the same diagnostic procedures used when the crown was initially placed. Necessary radiographs and periodontal tissue examinations should be made to rule out any periapical or periodontal disease such as bone loss, pocket formation, or furcation involvement (Figs. 1-19a to c).

Reasons to modify and preserve restorations

Quality of final result

The underlying premise of all procedures presented in this text is that the quality of the final modified restoration will be as good as or better than when it was initially placed. It should also meet the accepted criteria for any new restoration. The fractured facing shown (Fig. 1-20), could possibly be replaced with a new facing using one of the techniques described in the appropriate chapter. However, this would not correct the defects on the abutment tooth, such as the discoloration, the unesthetic margins, and the abnormal stress owing to faulty cantilever design.

Many considerations may enter into the decision to modify an existing restoration. First the dentist should consider whether his or her technical ability is equal to the task. Each dentist should always be expanding these technical abilities by proper training but one should not go beyond one's limitations. Some of the procedures presented here are very exacting and

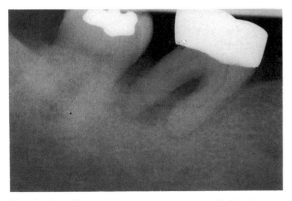

Fig. 1-19a Excessive bone loss around distal root.

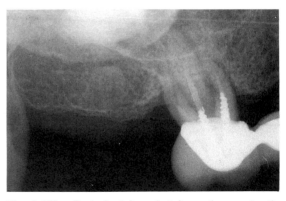

Fig. 1-19b Periodontal pocket formation on tooth with an existing bridge.

require close attention to detail, while others are somewhat less technique-sensitive.

Where laboratory procedures are involved, it is essential that the laboratory technician is capable of doing what is required. Before performing unusual procedures, it is best to check with the laboratory to be certain the necessary steps can be accomplished.

An existing restoration may be esthetically ideal but have a correctable defect in another area. For various reasons, it is possible that a complete remake of such a restoration might not be as ideal esthetically. This can be a compelling reason to save the restoration, if possible, without jeopardizing the long-term prognosis of the tooth.

When a component of an extensive restoration has a defect but remaking it would also require remaking many more components, it may be desirable to modify and preserve the existing restoration. For example, a multiple-unit broken connector fixed bridge may have acquired a correctable defect in the porcelain of one unit. While this correction would be essentially the same procedure as that done on a single unit, the remake of this restoration would be considerably more complicated, expensive, and risky.

Cost can be a factor as well. A patient may be unable to afford to have a restoration remade, or may need other more critical treatment, and

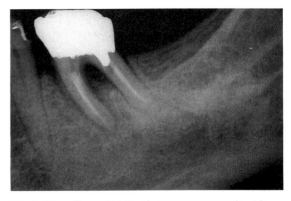

Fig. 1-19c Furcation involvement on a tooth with an existing crown.

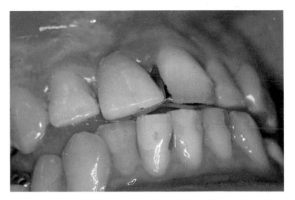

Fig. 1-20 Anterior cantilever bridge with broken facing that is not correctable due to defects related to the retainer.

cannot afford to have it all done at the present time. Modifying the restoration may save it either permanently or as a long-term temporary until the patient can afford to have it remade. When done as a long-term temporary, it must be clearly explained to the patient that this is not a permanent restoration. In no case should a dentist retain an existing restoration that by most standards should be remade.

Practical considerations

Since many people have dental insurance, dentists cannot ignore third-party involvement. Factors in the patient's insurance policies, such as annual maximum payments, waiting periods, or other time limitations, need to be taken into account in treatment planning. Phased treatment allows a patient to maximize insurance benefits and should be considered when it will not jeopardize the final result. However, when a treatment delay would lead to additional destruction of healthy tissue, modification of the existing restoration on a temporary basis may allow treatment to be staggered and thereby enable the patient to gain more of his fair share of insurance benefits. Other factors such as the patient's age and medical history may shift the treatment decision from remaking a restoration to modifying and preserving it.

The time involved in many modifications will be less than that required to make a new restoration. However, some modifications will take more time than creating and fitting a new restoration. This additional time will be justified when the overall benefits of saving a restoration outweigh the benefits of making a new one. In such a case, the dentist will usually be entitled to additional compensation commensurate with the added treatment time.

The final consideration is the number of modifications that can be justified to save one restoration. A tooth could conceivably have several correctable defects that on an individual basis could be corrected and give an excellent long-term prognosis. However, when added together, it may well be in the patient's best interest to make a new restoration that will be free of any of the defects. There is a limit to the number of modifications that can be made to a restoration without seriously compromising it. Good clinical judgment must be exercised in determining when that limit has been reached and which is the best course of treatment.

References

1. Challenges for the Eighties. National Institute of Dental Research—Long Range Research Plan, 1983.
2. Challenges for the Eighties. National Institute of Dental Research—Long Range Research Plan, 1983.
3. Moffa, J.P. Alternative dental casting alloys. D. Clin. N. Am. 27:733–746, 1983.
4. Leinfelder, K.F. Composite resins. D. Clin. N. Am. 29:359–372, 1985.
5. Jordan, R.E., et al. D. Clin. N. Am. 29:341–358, 1985.

Chapter 2

Removal of Existing Restorations

The removal of crowns and bridges has always been a challenging problem. A previously cemented restoration may need to be removed for any of the following reasons:

1. Marginal leakage and/or development of caries
2. Loss of interproximal contact due to drifting of teeth
3. Porcelain fracture that cannot be repaired in the mouth
4. Dissatisfaction with the esthetics of a porcelain-fused-to-metal restoration (Among other things, this can result from poor shade selection initially or from the surrounding teeth having changed shade over time.)
5. Perforation of the occlusal surface (due to wear) that cannot be corrected in the mouth
6. Post-cementation endodontics that weakened the coronal portion of the tooth such that a buildup and new crown is now needed
7. Casting that has been temporarily cemented
8. Casting that binds and is firmly affixed to the preparation upon try-in

Whenever a crown or bridge needs to be removed, *the most important consideration must be safety to the patient and prevention of damage to the remaining tooth structure as well as pulpal and periodontal tissues.* This point cannot be overemphasized and is the basis for the techniques presented here. Of secondary concern should be prevention of damage to the existing restoration, which is frequently unim-

portant since the restoration will often be remade anyway. However, even where it is desirable to save the existing restoration, such as during temporary cementation or try-in, sacrificing the casting is more often justified than is risking damage to the tooth. It is useless to have an undamaged crown or bridge in one's hand and no tooth on which to cement it because poor removal methods caused irreparable damage to the tooth and led to its extraction. *A new restoration for a given tooth can always be fabricated as long as that tooth is still restorable.*

Removal of a cast restoration, whether permanently or temporarily cemented, or just bound prior to cementation, requires force. If the force is too great or is misdirected, damage to the tooth can ensue. To reduce the possibility of damage, the force applied to remove the restoration should be directed as closely as possible in the long axis of the preparation. Before the dentist attempts to remove a cast restoration, several other questions should be raised.

1. *Did the dentist in question originally seat the restoration?* If so, he or she would have the advantage of knowing the unusual features of the design of the preparation relating to line of draw, retentive features, and so forth. Working casts may still be available, and could prove invaluable.

2. *Are there auxiliary retentive features such as grooves, boxes, or pins, which may complicate the removal of the casting?* Here the existence of the working casts may make the differ-

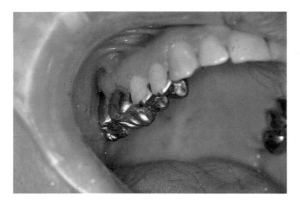

Fig. 2-1 Facial view of partial veneer and full crowns on maxillary arch.

ence between success and failure of the procedure, particularly in terms of the choice of method. In the absence of casts, one should assume there will be some irregularities in the preparation when applying force (Fig. 2-1).

3. *Does the tooth have a pin-retained buildup or some type of a post buildup?* If a post is present, is it separate from the crown, or is it part of it? While these questions may be impossible to answer unless the dentist asking them did the restoration, their answers are absolutely critical to a successful removal.

4. *Post or no post, has the tooth undergone endodontic therapy?* If so, the tooth will be more susceptible to damage from forces likely to be exerted during removal of the restoration, because so much more tooth structure has already been removed to gain access to the canal. This is particularly true in cases where endodontic therapy was performed after the crown was originally cemented.

5. *Is it desirable to save the crown for rece-mentation?* For example, the crown may have been temporarily cemented and now needs to be removed so it can be permanently cemented. Another common situation occurs when one retainer of a fixed bridge has become loose and the other is still tight. If the second abutment can be removed without damaging the tooth, all that may be necessary is recementation. This would depend on the reason the first retainer lost retention. Occasionally the only reason was

poor handling of the cement, with no real defect in the retentive aspects of the restoration itself or the preparation.

The answers to the aforementioned questions will be helpful in determining how to remove an existing crown or bridge. The following should be considered whenever possible:

1. Working casts of the preparation
2. Radiographs, especially those taken during an endodontic procedure, which show the preparation (The general dentist should not hesitate to request these from the endodontist.)
3. The dentist's recollection of the preparation if he or she did it, as well as any notes recorded in the patient's treatment record.
4. Photographs taken during the procedure

Many devices and techniques have been advocated for use in removing existing cast restorations.[1] Most of these are detrimental to the integrity of the casting and are dangerous to the tooth. Many of these methods place unnecessary and potentially injurious stresses on the tooth. The methods advocated in this text place minimal stress on the tooth, and are safe when properly used. Again, the primary and overriding principle is that *no restoration is worth the loss of a useable tooth, regardless of how much laboratory and clinical time and expense was involved.*

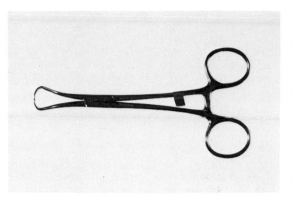

Fig. 2-2 Backhaus clamp for removal of temporary crowns.

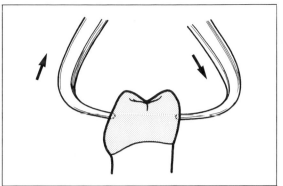

Fig. 2-3 Backhaus clamp engaging temporary crown and applying force in a gingival direction lingually and an occlusal direction facially.

Removal of temporary restorations

An integral part of the procedure for constructing fixed prosthodontic restorations is the use of temporary restorations while the final ones are being made in the laboratory. These may take several different forms, depending on the situation at hand and the individual dentist's preferences. Some of the more common methods are: *(1)* indirect custom acrylic, *(2)* direct custom acrylic, *(3)* preformed metal (either as manufactured or relined with acrylic), and *(4)* preformed polycarbonate.

Regardless of the method used to arrive at such a temporary restoration, eventually the restoration must be removed in order to proceed with the treatment at a subsequent appointment. The requirements of this type of restoration are conflicting ones. First, it must fit well enough and be cemented with a strong enough temporary cement to allow the patient to function normally without the restoration coming loose between appointments. However, it should not be so difficult to remove that it causes the patient discomfort. Usually, the temporary restoration will need to be removed without using anesthesia, so that when the final restoration is being tried in, proper adjustment of the occlusion can be made.

Method

Step 1

The instrument of choice for this method is the Backhaus clamp.* It is uniquely suited to the procedure and allows temporary crowns to be removed atraumatically (Fig. 2-2).

Step 2

Place a 4 × 4 gauze in the back of the mouth to prevent possible aspiration of the restoration.

Step 3

Position the beaks of the clamp near the middle of the facial and lingual surfaces of the restoration if it is a full crown. If it is a partial veneer crown or onlay, position the clamp beaks at whatever spots will allow for engagement of the temporary prosthesis on two opposing surfaces, without danger of contacting a finish line.

Step 4

Break the cement seal using a rocking motion with moderate force in an occlusal direction on one surface and in the gingival direction on the other (Fig. 2-3).

*Union Broach Co., Long Island City, N.Y.

31

Removal of temporarily cemented permanent crowns

Occasionally, it is advantageous to seat a permanent crown or bridge on a temporary basis. Some of the following situations may be indications to do so:

1. The patient may want to view and evaluate the esthetics in his or her own environment, such as with family members, and with more natural types of lighting than are available in the office, such as sunlight.

2. The dentist may think that the occlusion is questionable and wish to have the patient functioning on the restoration for a period prior to permanently committing both himself or herself and the patient to the occlusal scheme.

3. In the case of a bridge, the question of pontic form sometimes arises. Often, an old bridge will have had a saddle-shaped gingival surface. Since this design is hygienically undesirable, the new bridge will usually have a different design and the patient may have difficulty getting used to it. The fact that the patient knows that this is a "trial" period and that changes can still be made often makes it easier for the patient to accept this change and ultimately to adjust to it.

4. Temporary cementation of a multiple-unit anterior restoration also allows evaluation of the restoration from a phonetics standpoint. Too often restorations involving the maxillary anterior teeth give patients speech problems. Certain sounds are now more difficult or impossible. Examples might be "f" or "ph" where the incisal length of the central incisors is too short or "th" where the lingual surface is not correctly contoured. This kind of error can be avoided very easily by using a temporary restoration which has been produced by using a diagnostic waxup rather than the patient's original tooth form. This temporary restoration can be adjusted and modified as indicated while the patient functions routinely. When the final restoration is accomplished, a duplication of this form is all that is necessary. The relationship of anterior tooth form to certain professional activities such as playing brass or woodwind instruments should also be considered.

Any permanent casting which is temporarily cemented may be difficult to remove without damaging the crown. This point must be understood by both the dentist and patient. Before any casting is cemented on a temporary basis, the dentist must have a general idea of the way the restoration will be removed when it is time to permanently cement it. This plan must encompass not only the importance of preventing damage to the restoration, but also the principle of safety to the tooth and its supporting structures. One must recognize a fine line here: We want the crown to stay in place while the patient functions on it, just as it would if it were permanently cemented, yet we need to be able to remove it easily later. These are conflicting requirements, which in actual practice may be impossible to satisfy in all cases. This danger must be understood ahead of time by all concerned.

In the case of a relatively ideal preparation, temporary cement can provide sufficient retention to make removal of the crown very difficult. Conversely, a concern in temporary cementation is the lack of retention in some cases. If the crown comes out between appointments, the patient could swallow, aspirate, damage, or lose it. The most serious of these possibilities is aspiration into the bronchial tree. Clinical judgment is critical and the dentist must decide in each individual case whether the benefits of cementing single units on a temporary basis outweigh the potential hazards, particularly in the case of single units which are more likely to come loose and can be aspirated more easily than a bridge.

It has been shown that with the same cement, a cast crown will require more force to remove than an acrylic crown. This should be considered when deciding which cement to use.

If a permanent restoration will be cemented temporarily, this should be planned for in the waxing phase. Removal buttons should be added to the lingual surface of a single unit (Fig. 2-4). This will allow the dentist a method of relatively safe removal of the casting when it is time to permanently cement it. The instrument for the actual removal is a matter of the practitioner's choice, but often the choice is a reverse mallet (Figs. 2-5a and b) or a periodontal scaler. The button can be removed with appropriate rotary instruments and the casting can be polished before final cementation.

One word of caution regarding this removal method: Since it is necessary that the removal button be on an external surface, it is well away from the central axis of the preparation. This means that there will be a vector of force acting in a lateral direction on the preparation. Consequently, care should be taken to avoid applying too much force, which could cause the remaining tooth structure to fracture.

Three removal methods can be used for temporarily cemented restorations:

1. If a removal button has been placed, then the reverse mallet is effective (Figs. 2-5a and b).
2. If no button has been placed the Backhaus clamp is often the best choice, provided that opposing surfaces are metal, since porcelain is not engaged by the beaks (Fig. 2-2).
3. The Richwill Crown and Bridge Remover* can be useful (Fig. 2-7a).

Each of these is discussed later in this chapter.

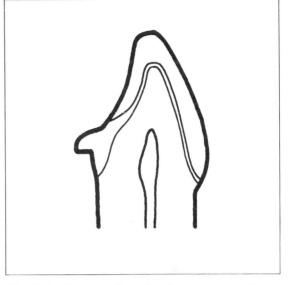

Fig. 2-4 Cross-section of anterior crown with removal button on lingual.

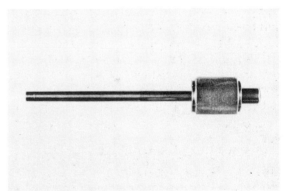
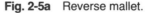

Fig. 2-5a Reverse mallet.

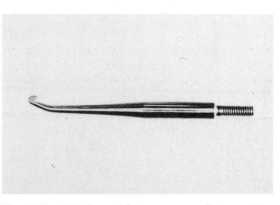

Fig. 2-5b Attachment for reverse mallet used for crown removal.

*Richwill Laboratories, Orange, Calif.

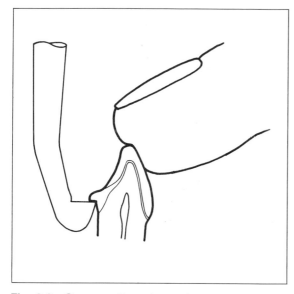

Fig. 2-6 Cross-section of anterior crown with reverse mallet engaging removal button and finger on facial surface.

lingually to aid in resisting the lateral vector of force that will be applied by the mallet when engaging the removal button (Fig. 2-6).

Step 5

Engage the tip of the reverse mallet under the removal button with the long axis of the handle in line with the long axis of the preparation.

Step 6

Slide the "hammer" along the handle in several short, quick strokes until the crown loosens. Depending on the degree of parallelism of the preparation and the type of cement used, the crown should be removed in a few strokes. If not, carefully consider the risks and benefits of increasing the force.

Method: Reverse mallet

Step 1

Form removal button during the waxup phase. The proper size for this button will allow for sound engagement of an instrument under it, but should not be so large or of such a contour that patient irritation occurs.

Step 2

Carefully examine the working cast to assess the amount of force that can be applied on the button without fracturing the preparation.

Step 3

Place a 4 × 4 gauze in the back of the mouth to prevent aspiration of the restoration.

Step 4

Have the dental assistant place a finger on the facial surface of the restoration and apply force

Method: Richwill crown and bridge remover

One device that can be very effective in removing a casting without damaging the restoration or the tooth is the Richwill Crown and Bridge Remover.[3] This method is based on a principle of adhesion, and results in the restoration being reusable. The success of this method depends on equal and opposite force being applied to the two opposing teeth if the material contacts only one tooth in each arch (Figs. 2-7a and b). It is "assumed" that the crown we are trying to remove has less retention than the one on the opposing tooth, if one is present. This assumption, which may not be defensible in some cases, is addressed below.

Step 1

The remover comes two to a sealed plastic packet. Place the packet into 145°F water for one to two minutes to condition it. The tempering bath of a hydrocolloid conditioner is adequate, as is a water bath similar to that used for softening waxes and border-molding-compounds in prosthetic procedures. One can tell if the material is properly softened by attempting

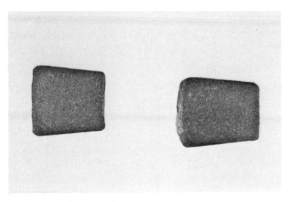

Fig. 2-7a Richwill Crown and Bridge Remover.

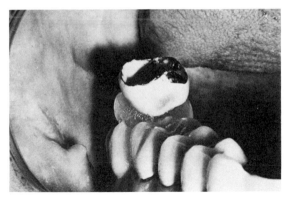

Fig. 2-7b Crown after removal still attached to Richwill Crown and Bridge Remover.

to compress it slightly with the fingers. It will allow for some compression while in the untempered state but it cannot be compressed at all with the fingers.

Step 2

While the remover is being conditioned, examine the teeth in the area in both arches and their restorations. The opposing teeth need to be healthy and periodontally solid. Ideally, they should be free of crowns, and have only relatively conservative silver amalgams or no restorations at all. A full denture or partial denture in the opposite arch may preclude the dentist from successfully using this method.

If crowns are present, the patient should be advised of the possibility that such crowns could be removed during the procedure if they have minimal retention. One could argue that if this occurs, the opposing crown was probably not adequately retentive and may need replacement. After the fact, however, this kind of explanation is clearer to the dentist than to the patient. A modification of the standard method will be described below.

Step 3

The patient now needs to be instructed as to their part of the procedure, since the success of this technique is largely dependent on patient cooperation. They should be told that they will be closing into the remover material, holding steady for about 10 seconds, then opening with a quick movement. The patient will feel considerable resistance to this movement.

Step 4

After conditioning the remover and instructing the patient, tie dental floss around the remover as a precaution against accidental aspiration or swallowing.

Step 5

Place the individual remover in hot water for a few seconds. Avoid touching it when it is out of the plastic packet, since it is extremely sticky. Blow off excess moisture, but do not actually dry it. Place it over the crown using an instrument such as a small spoon imbedded 1 or 2 mm into the remover.

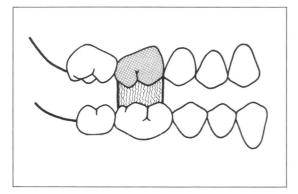

Fig. 2-8 Compressed Richwill Crown and Bridge Remover attached to crown to be removed and opposing tooth.

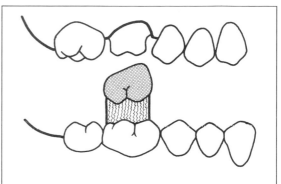

Fig. 2-9 Richwill Crown and Bridge Remover still attached to crown after removal.

Step 6

Instruct the patient to close, compressing the remover about two-thirds of its previous height, and hold that position for 10 seconds (Fig. 2-8). In the case of a molar or premolar crown, the patient should close in centric position, while for anterior crowns patients should close in a protrusive position.

Step 7

Have the patient open with a quick, forceful movement. If the crown comes off the preparation, it will remain attached to the remover, which will itself be attached to the opposing tooth (Fig. 2-9). Detach the crown and remover from the opposing tooth, then detach the crown from the remover. Using a suitable instrument, clean off any remnants of the remover from the crown and the opposing tooth.

If the crown does not come off the first time, it will be necessary to repeat this procedure using a new remover each time. Frequently, additional attempts will successfully remove the crown.

Step 8

As an alternative method for situations where the dentist thinks there is a possibility of removing an opposing single crown, it is usually very helpful to form the material in a pyramid shape.

Position the remover with the apex of the pyramid toward the crown to be removed, and the base toward the opposing arch. The remover will contact only the crown to be removed in its arch, but will contact several different teeth in the opposing arch, thus distributing the force to teeth other than just the one with the crown in the opposing arch. The dentist will need to carefully watch the patient's closure and prevent him or her from closing so far as to spread the material out and contact other teeth in the arch of the crown to be removed.

Removal of a temporarily cemented permanent bridge

The Richwill Crown and Bridge Remover can be used to remove a temporarily cemented bridge using the aforementioned principles and the method just described. The only variation is that normally it is best to place a separate remover on each retainer (Figs. 2-10a and b).

In other situations, the proper temporary cement can be the dentist's best aid. Opotow Trial Cement* can be effectively used for short-term temporary cementation of bridges. It is usually adequate for retention of the bridge and re-

*Teledyne Getz, Elk Grove Village, Ill.

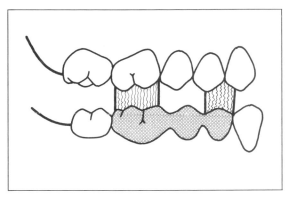

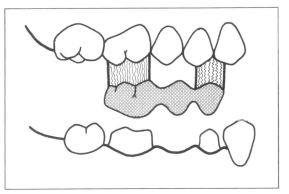

Fig. 2-10a Two compressed Richwill Crown and Bridge Removers attached to bridge to be removed and opposing teeth.

Fig. 2-10b Richwill Crown and Bridge Removers still attached to bridge after removal.

moval can easily be accomplished with a small piece of gauze. This cement forms a soft gasket and never really hardens. It is not recommended for single units, owing to lack of retention.

Frequently in the case of a bridge, it is possible to accomplish the removal by taking advantage of the connectors. Either dental floss looped around the underside of a connector or a reverse mallet type of remover engaging the underside of the connector can be used. This device can be very hazardous and should never be used in cases of great retention or where the dentist is unfamiliar with the preparation. For more details on use of this technique, please refer to the section on removal of a permanent bridge with one loose retainer, later in this chapter.

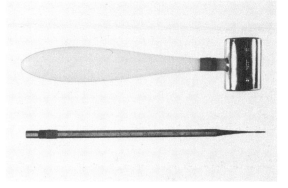

Fig. 2-11 Straight chisel and mallet.

Removal of a crown at try-in

Removal of a crown at the try-in stage that binds on the preparation or interproximally can be a delicate procedure. The quickest method for removal uses a straight chisel, and *very gentle* tapping with a mallet (Fig. 2-11). The chisel is placed on the mesial of the casting just below the mesial contact.

With the chisel pointed toward the occlusal in a direction as near to parallel with the line of draw of the preparation as possible (Fig. 2-12),

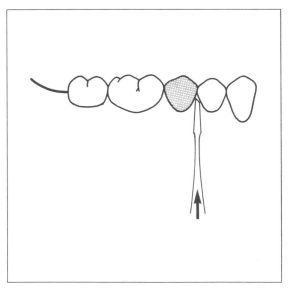

Fig. 2-12 Straight chisel on mesial surface of crown being tried in showing proper direction of force.

one or two light taps will usually loosen the casting. The casting should then be removable with the fingers and a piece of gauze. The chisel needs to be in the direction of the line of draw of the crown to prevent fracture of the tooth or damage to the crown (Fig. 2-13).

It is important to use a 4×4 gauze in the back of the mouth to prevent aspirating or swallowing the crown if it should suddenly come off. Also, having an assistant place a finger lightly on the occlusal surface as the mallet is used will prevent the crown from coming off in an uncontrolled fashion. If a few light taps do not loosen the crown, employ another method. *Again, the most important consideration is preservation of the patient's dentition and oral health, not the preservation of a restoration.*

If this method fails to remove a crown which is binding, using the Richwill remover as previously described will usually accomplish the task.

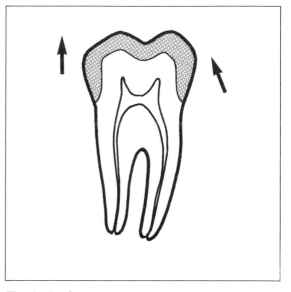

Fig. 2-13 Cross-section of tooth showing correct and incorrect directions of force. Correct direction parallels long axis of tooth.

Removal of a permanent bridge with one loose retainer

Occasionally, one retainer of a fixed bridge will come loose while the other one remains retentive. If a failure of the cement bond occurs with a single crown, the restoration will simply come off and the patient will seek the services of the dentist. The danger in the case of a fixed bridge, however, is that often the restoration will not actually come out because the other retainer is keeping it in place—and the patient is unaware of the problem. As often happens, the abutment preparation under the loose retainer becomes slowly but surely decalcified, owing to the constant long-term ingress of fluids. It is not uncommon for this tooth to be lost, or at the very least, to require endodontic therapy and a post to save it before the new bridge is made.

The first sign of trouble sometimes is pain as the pulp becomes involved. When a patient complains that a bridge feels loose, careful evaluation is essential. However, by the time the patient becomes aware of the problem, the damage is usually extensive.

When the cement seal is lost and the bridge remains cemented to the other abutment, bacteria and oral fluids can get under the casting and remain relatively undisturbed. In a comparatively short period, the minerals in the tooth can be dissolved and the tooth will become very soft. This can be the case even though the tooth appears normal at first glance except for a little stain. More careful examination often reveals a tooth soft enough for an explorer to penetrate completely through it, or at least to bend the tooth as if it were leather. When this is the case, the procedure here involves removal of the other, still cemented, retainer without damage to that tooth. Then a new fixed bridge will be necessary, after appropriate treatment of the demineralized tooth.

Because of the potential damage of such a situation, the following procedure is recommended when a patient complains of a loose bridge: Place an explorer under the connector

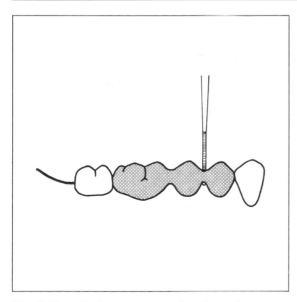

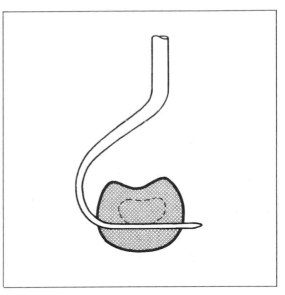

Fig. 2-14a Explorer on gingival surface of connector of fixed bridge applying light force in an occlusal direction to check for loose retainer.

Fig. 2-14b Cross-section of explorer on gingival surface of connector of fixed bridge.

between the suspected unit and the pontic, and apply light pressure in an occlusal direction (Figs. 2-14a and b). This is a good procedure to follow at recall appointments for all fixed bridge patients. Then apply force in an apical direction with a finger on the occlusal surface of the suspected unit. Using magnification, observe the gingival margin for the movement of fluids, and the formation of small bubbles (Fig. 2-15).

It may be desirable to remove the bridge without damaging it. This is viable only if the looseness is discovered at a very early stage and no damage has yet occurred to the tooth. There are two methods that can be used:

Method: Richwill Crown and Bridge Remover

This method has been described previously in this chapter, in the section on removal of temporarily cemented permanent crowns. The only modification is that care should be taken to place the remover only over the retainer that is still cemented, to avoid the lateral vector of force

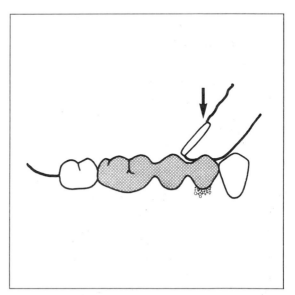

Fig. 2-15 Force applied gingivally on loose retainer of a fixed bridge. Note bubbles at the gingival margin of the loose retainer.

which would develop if the remover were to be placed over the pontic or the loose retainer. In this case, the cemented retainer is treated as though it were a single unit.

Method: Reverse mallet

The reverse mallet can be used to remove a permanently cemented bridge when one retainer has become loose. Normally there is no justification for using this method to remove a bridge when both retainers are still permanently cemented. It should not be used to attempt to remove a single unit except for one that is temporarily cemented and has a removal button. It is simply too hard to apply an occlusally directed force when the contour of most single units does not provide for any undercuts such as are provided for by a bridge connector or a removal button. There are potential hazards that must be understood by the dentist and then explained to the patient. The patient must understand the risks and choose to accept some responsibility if something untoward happens. The primary risks are: *(1)* pulpal and periapical irritation; *(2)* gingival irritation; *(3)* damage to the bridge; and *(4)* fracture of the abutment tooth.

The sudden and repetitive forces required to break the cement seal on the remaining abutment tooth are potentially traumatic to the pulp, particularly the vessels entering and leaving the apical foramina. While this effect is certainly minimal, it should not be discounted entirely when added to the previous insults of tooth preparation, impressions, and the temporary phase in which the temporary restoration may have come loose at one point.

Gingival irritation can be caused by improper placement of the tip of the reverse mallet in between the connector and the tissue. While this will often be caused by carelessness of the dentist, it is often an unavoidable result of the initial contour of the restoration.

Damage to the bridge will occur most often where porcelain is fused to the metal near the connector. If this happens, it may be possible to correct the problem in the laboratory by baking porcelain in the area. Usually, however, this will not result in a satisfactory restoration. The entire porcelain will most likely need to be replaced, which will necessitate stripping all the porcelain off the coping and rebaking. In both cases, it will be necessary to temporize the teeth while the laboratory work is being done. Before removal is attempted the patient should understand that the bridge may need to be remade.

Damage can also occur to the metal part of the bridge, but this will almost always be limited to minor scratches that can be polished off. Any substantial change in the metal occurring during removal, such as a bent margin, will necessitate remaking the restoration.

Finally, fracture of the abutment tooth is the ultimate disaster. This is probably the most common untoward result of using the reverse mallet, and is the reason the authors advocate extreme caution in the use of this instrument. A fracture can range in severity from a small chip to one in which the pulp is exposed, or one so severe the tooth cannot be restored. This latter possibility is even more likely in a tooth that has had endodontic treatment without a post. Of particular concern is the tooth that has had endodontic treatment through the existing restoration. Only in very rare instances should this method of removal be attempted in such a case.

Step 1

Carefully examine current radiographs of the tooth in question, paying particular attention to the direction of its long axis. If a cast of the preparation is available, examine it for the line of draw and general form. This latter aid will not usually be available, but may be in a case where the same dentist recently cemented the restoration.

Step 2

If necessary, anesthetize the area. Place the proper reverse mallet tip under the connector next to the cemented retainer. This is usually best accomplished from the lingual aspect, but can also be done from the facial aspect (Fig. 2-16). Several different tip sizes and shapes are available and the chosen one should be the one least likely to cause tissue trauma, while at the same time providing a good purchase on the restoration (Figs. 2-17a and b). Occasionally, it may be necessary to reshape the tip.

Step 3

Have the assistant place a finger on the loose retainer, so that the force applied by the reverse mallet will not cause the bridge to rotate occlusally, and apply a torque to the cemented abutment.

Step 4

Engage the tip of the reverse mallet under the connector with the long axis of the handle in line with the long axis of the preparation.

Step 5

Slide the "hammer" along the handle with several short, quick strokes until the retainer is loosened. Depending on the degree of parallelism of the preparation and the type of cement used, it should be removed in a few strokes. If not, further attempts by increasing the force should be carefully considered by weighing the benefits against the risks.

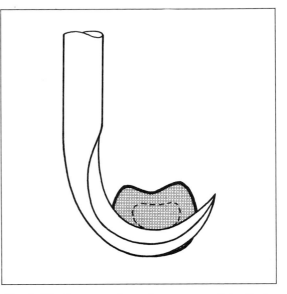

Fig. 2-16 Cross-section of reverse mallet attachment on gingival surface of connector of fixed bridge.

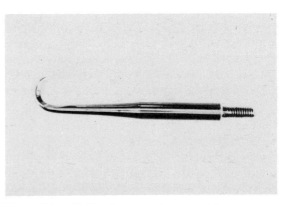

Fig. 2-17a Sickle-shaped attachment for reverse mallet.

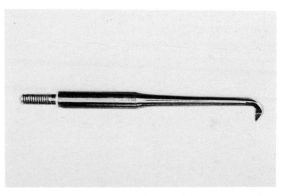

Fig. 2-17b Serrated attachment for reverse mallet.

Removal of a permanently cemented restoration which is to be remade

The following technique should be the most common method used for removal of permanently cemented restorations because:

1. It is seldom that the existing restoration will be reused. It usually has some defect, and if not, will often be damaged during removal.
2. It most safely satisfies the principle of protecting the remaining tooth structure, which is of paramount importance, rather than the restoration.
3. It is usually the least traumatic to the patient.

Once the decision has been made to remove the restoration without saving it for reuse, this is the only technique the authors recommend.

Method: When an impression is yet to be made

Step 1

Study radiographs carefully. Any obvious pathology such as periapical or periodontal defects should be noted, and it should be determined whether it would be better to treat the pathology before or after removal of the restoration. For example, it may be best to do an endodontic procedure while the old crown is still on the preparation, while a periodontal lesion or cervical caries would often be better treated with the old crown out of the way. The presence of a post in the canal will require special treatment, as described later in this chapter.

Step 2

Clinically examine the casting. If it is a partial veneer crown of any kind, it will have grooves, boxes, or pins which are an integral part of the casting and which will also require special care, as described later in this chapter in a section on special situations. The working casts of the case that show the preparation itself can make the difference between a successful and a disastrous removal.

Step 3

Anesthetize the tooth if necessary. In the case of a vital tooth, this is usually advisable.

Step 4

Using a round end cross-cut fissure bur such as a no. 1558, or a round bur such as a no. 4, begin at the most accessible margin of the crown, usually the facial margin. Make a cut through the casting to the cement film (Fig. 2-18). Magnification, such as $2\times$ or $4\times$ loops, is very advisable here and will make it much easier to identify the cement by its contrast in color with the gold. If the crown is porcelain, make the initial groove with a diamond until the gold coping is reached; then switch to a carbide bur. Continue the groove up the facial surface, across the occlusal and down the lingual, until only a band of about 2 mm is left connecting the halves at the lingual gingival margin of the casting (Figs. 2-19a to c). In this manner, there will be less chance of the patient aspirating or swallowing one of the halves. The ideal result is a groove through the casting with cement at the base of the groove, with no groove in the underlying tooth structure (Fig. 2-20).

Step 5

Place a 4×4 gauze in the back of the mouth to prevent the patient from aspirating or swallowing the restoration after it is removed from the tooth.

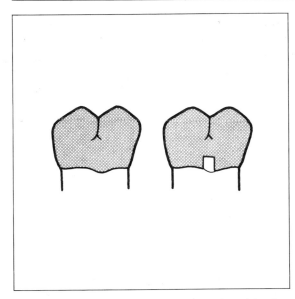

Fig. 2-18 Crown to be removed on left and beginning groove at gingival margin on facial surface, exposing cement film, as shown on right.

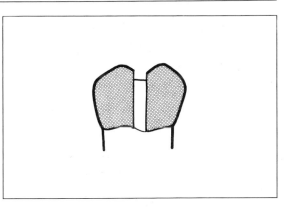

Fig. 2-19a Groove extending up the facial surface to occlusal surface.

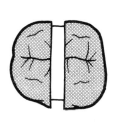

Fig. 2-19b Groove extending across occlusal surface to lingual surface.

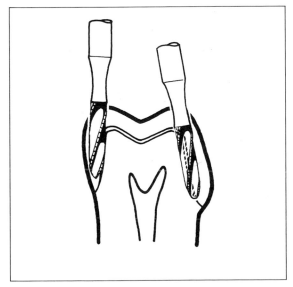

Fig. 2-20 Bur on lingual surface at correct depth. Bur on facial surface has penetrated too deeply, resulting in an unnecessary groove in the wall of the preparation.

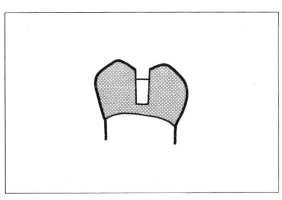

Fig. 2-19c Groove extending down lingual surface leaving 2 mm of uncut casting.

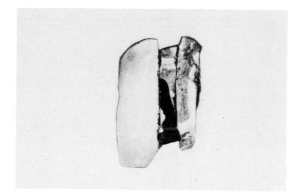

Fig. 2-21 Crown after removal, with porcelain having broken off one-half of coping.

Step 6

Place a large spoon excavator or similar instrument in the groove and use one side of the groove as a fulcrum to apply a controlled force to the opposite half of the casting. Usually the cement bond will quickly break, then the process can be reversed by applying pressure to the first half of the restoration to break its bond. In the case of porcelain-fused-to-metal crowns, the porcelain will usually break off one part of the coping which then allows for ease in bending the remaining metal (Fig. 2-21).

The series of photographs (Figs. 2-22a to d) show this technique applied in a clinical situation, emphasizing the importance of carefully and neatly approaching the procedure. The an-

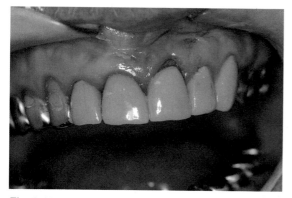

Fig. 2-22a Four anterior crowns to be removed.

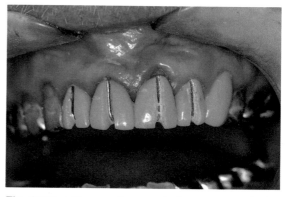

Fig. 2-22b Proper placement of grooves on facial surface through porcelain to gold.

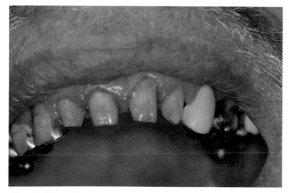

Fig. 2-22c Preparations with crowns removed.

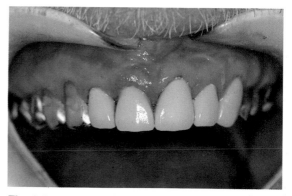

Fig. 2-22d New crowns in place.

terior crowns are being removed with virtually no damage to the underlying tooth structure by cutting off the old crowns, rather than applying force in a less controlled manner as is often done. Until the preparations are visible, as in Fig. 2-22c, the dentist has no way of knowing which of these teeth might be irreparably damaged by injudicious use of force.

Step 7

If the cement bond does not easily break, cut a trough between the casting and the occlusal surface of the preparation using a small round bur, preferably at the expense of the casting. Then, an instrument can be placed into this groove and force applied in an occlusal direction.

Method: Impression already made, finish lines of preparation must not be altered

Occasionally, a permanent crown will be seated on a temporary basis while a new crown to replace it is being made in the laboratory. Perhaps at the try-in, the crown had an improperly fitting margin and a new impression was made for a second crown. Then, as an interim restoration, the first crown was cemented temporarily, rather than a more customary acrylic or preformed metal temporary. Whatever the reason for this action, there are instances when it is impossible to remove this crown at the subsequent appointment when the time comes to cement the new restoration.

If the usual means for removal referred to earlier are successful, there is no problem. The first approach should be to use the Richwill remover, discussed under the section on removal of temporarily cemented permanent crowns earlier in this chapter. Most of the time, this will be successful. If it is not, it will be necessary to cut this crown off, but without damaging the finish line of the preparation, since the new crown which is about to be seated was made on a die representing the existing finish lines. The procedure is described for a full

crown, but can be adapted to partial veneer crowns as well. For a crown that has grooves or boxes for retention, special care must be taken to not damage the tooth. This problem is addressed in the next section of this chapter. If there is any doubt as to the safety to the tooth, one should always follow the course with the least potential for damage to the tooth. The following steps will achieve this:

Step 1

Use a no. 1558 carbide bur in a high-speed handpiece and start a groove in the most accessible surface of the crown, usually the facial, just exposing the cement line. If the crown is porcelain-fused-to-metal, use a diamond stone to cut through the porcelain until the metal is reached, then switch to the carbide bur. This groove must end at least 1 to 2 mm from the margin of the crown. In this variation of the method described previously, it is imperative that the finish line of the preparation be untouched by the bur.

Step 2

Continue the groove up the initial surface of the crown, across the occlusal and down the opposite side of the crown to a point no less than 1 to 2 mm from the margin again. The crown should have a groove which exposes the cement line from one side to the other except for two narrow bands of metal adjacent to the margins on opposite sides of the tooth (Figs. 2-23a and b). This is more critical than in the standard version of this method because the mode of fracture of the cement bond will be the actual movement of the occlusal portions of the casting mesially and distally. This will be impossible if even the slightest connection of metal exists between the two halves of the casting at any point other than near the margins.

Step 3

Place a spoon excavator or other similar instrument in the groove on the occlusal or incisal

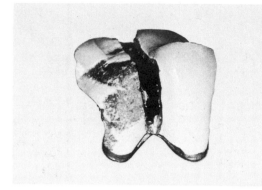

Fig. 2-23a Crown after removal with uncut facial margin.

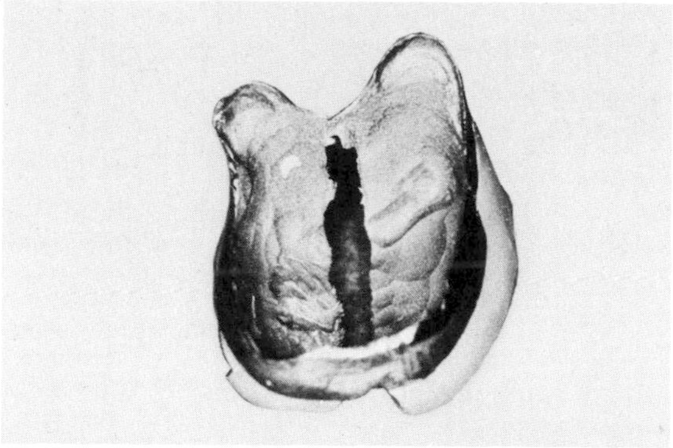

Fig. 2-23b Crown after removal with uncut lingual margin.

surface and gently put pressure on the two halves of the crown to force them away from each other. This should break the cement seal and allow the crown to be removed with a spoon or Backhaus clamp. Ideally, the underlying tooth should be undamaged, so that the finish line is complete and accurate.

Removal of permanently cemented restorations with special features

Most of the aforementioned methods will prove adequate and safe in the vast majority of cases, since the removal of most castings involves the full crown design. Occasionally, however, the crown preparation embodies one or more special features such as:

1. Partial veneer crowns incorporating the typical mesial and distal grooves for auxiliary retention
2. Pin-retained castings which will have either pins cast of the parent alloy or high-tensile pins to which the parent alloy was cast
3. Telescope crowns in which one casting is cemented on top of another
4. Dowel cores or other endodontic posts
5. Inlays

Removal of partial veneer crowns

Since by definition these castings utilize auxiliary retention, the technique described previously, which involved making a cut through the casting to the cement line and then applying pressure to "open" the crown and break the cement seal, must be modified (Fig. 2-24). It is essential that the dentist know and appreciate the location and angulation of the grooves in different types of partial veneer crown preparations. For example, a three-quarter crown may present minimal problems as a cut made in a faciolingual direction would still permit the crown to be spread open without any adverse force applied at the grooves. This might not be the case with a seven-eighth crown, however, in which the facial groove would be the site of adverse forces if the crown were spread mesially and distally (Fig. 2-25), raising the risk of tooth fracture.

The solution is twofold. First, it is extremely helpful if the dentist has the working casts for reference, or at least can recall the preparation design. Second, one can assume the likely location of the grooves, and then apply limited force.

When that threshold is reached and no movement occurs, stop the application of spreading force and continue to cut another groove or extend the present groove farther. In these cases, there is no substitute for patience.

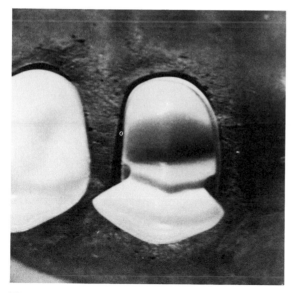

Fig. 2-24 Model of ideal three-quarter crown preparation.

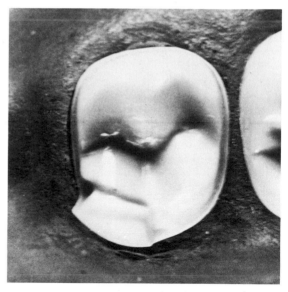

Fig. 2-25 Model of ideal seven-eighth crown preparation.

Keep in mind, that these typical examples could embody modifications such as boxes which could prevent resistance to movement and the subsequent application of potentially damaging forces.

Removal of pin-retained castings

Pin-retained restorations present some of the most perplexing problems when removal is needed. The reason is fairly simple, namely the presence of pins in the dentin. However, that does not make it easier to handle because often the dentist does not know the pins are present. Pins sometimes do not show up on radiographs owing to the curvature of the facial and lingual margins of the casting itself. Even if one pin is visible, others may not be (Fig. 2-26).

Here again, a firsthand knowledge of the preparation, the number, and the location of the pins is a tremendous asset. Without such knowledge, the dentist will have to make independent judgments with very limited information. Here it

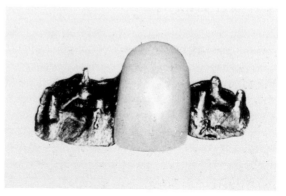

Fig. 2-26 Pin-retained casting.

is very important to warn the patient of potential risks, and the fact that, incongruous as it may seem, such a sophisticated design may well make it ultimately impossible to save the tooth.

Basically, the dentist must attempt to remove the casting in the presumed line of draw of the pins. One of the essential features of a casting with pin retention is that no displacement is possible in any direction other than the long axis of the pins themselves. Contrast this with the grooves or boxes of a partial veneer crown which allow for displacement in a direction away from the axial wall as well as along the line of draw. In this context, one must not confuse the term "pin-retained casting" with "pin-retained buildup," such as using TMS pins screwed into the dentin.[6]

Another feature of pin retention is that while there is a great resistance to lateral displacement, which is the kind of movement most likely to make a crown come loose in the mouth during function, there is considerably less retention along the long axis of the pins themselves. This can often work to the dentist's advantage, and makes this situation amenable to using the Richwill Crown and Bridge Remover. The bottom line in these cases is that unless the casting can be removed by a technique which applies force only in the long axis of the pins, it probably cannot be removed at all.

Another alternative which has limited success is to cut a groove along the gingival margin on either the facial or lingual surface, preferably both, and apply leverage between the dentin of the root and the gingival margin area of the casting. This method requires the presence of at least 1 to 2 mm of exposed tooth structure gingival to the old casting margin so that the new margin created by the groove will be in an acceptable location for the new crown. While this method may seem a bit radical and not in keeping with the basic principle of protecting the remaining tooth, we are assuming that if the crown cannot be removed, the tooth needs to be extracted anyway.

It is always possible—and will frequently be the best alternative—to make a horizontal cut through the gingival aspect of the crown, cutting off the pins and leaving them imbedded in the tooth structure. Then, with the old crown off, a decision will be made as to the prognosis of the tooth and the specific restorative method to be employed. It may be possible to drill new pinholes, but this is usually not advisable in terms of the future integrity of the tooth structure. More often than not, the tooth will need to be devitalized and a post placed into the canal.

Removal of telescope crowns

If the reader were to refer to the section of this chapter which details the method of making a cut through the casting until a cement line is visible, the problem of cutting off a telescope crown from its undercoping becomes obvious: When cutting through a crown seated on a dentin preparation, one first encounters the white cement, then if the cut is made too deep, the dentin is encountered. In both instances the dentist is at least aware of having passed through the casting, because of the difference in color. However, when cutting the superstructure of a telescope crown off of the gold coping underneath it, the cement line is reached and passed so quickly, that it often is not noticed. Then, the cut is again being made in a gold casting indistinguishable from the superstructure casting. The problem here is that it may not have been the intent to remove both parts, but to remove only the crown, and leave the coping cemented to the tooth.

The solution is clear: Make the cut carefully and patiently and watch for the ever-elusive cement line. Magnification, such as $2 \times$ or $4 \times$ loops, is essential.

Removal of crowns from dowel cores

The ability to remove a crown retained by a cast dowel core will usually depend on whether the crown is separate from the dowel core casting. For this reason *no crown which is retained by a dowel in the canal should ever be made integral with the dowel, but should always be a separate casting.* Consequently, it will be possible to remove the crown later without injuring the root of the tooth by attempting to remove the dowel.

If there is reason to believe that the crown and the dowel are one casting, a radiographic evaluation should be made of the structural integrity of the root and the apparent retentive features of the dowel such as length and degree of parallelism (Fig. 2-27). If the dentist has reason to question the retentive capabilities of the dowel but the root appears sound, he or she can attempt to remove it using the Richwill Crown

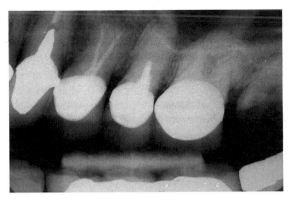

Fig. 2-27 Short dowel in cuspid.

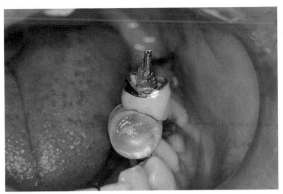

Fig. 2-28 Richwill remover still attached to dowel crown after removal.

and Bridge Remover, since the objective is to remove it in the long axis of the root (Fig. 2-28).

It will often be necessary to attempt to remove a crown which has a cast dowel in the canal without knowing whether it is a one- or two-piece restoration. In such a case, the following procedure should be followed:

Step 1

Cut the groove through the facial surface, as described in the technique for removing a crown from a natural tooth preparation. However, take the same precaution as discussed in the case of a telescope crown—carefully watch for the cement line, and immediately upon encountering it, do not cut any deeper. Make a wider groove than you would in removing a normally cemented crown so that it will be easier to detect the thin cement line.

Step 2

Once the cement line is encountered, extend the cut in both directions until the line is evident on the entire facial surface and most of the lingual surface, leaving only a small tag of gold connecting the two halves on the lingual at the margin area.

Step 3

Remove the crown as described earlier in this

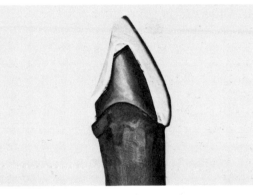

Fig. 2-29 Cross-section of ideal anterior porcelain-fused-to-metal crown and preparation.

chapter in the section on removal of a permanently cemented restoration which is to be remade.

Step 4

If, however, the casting is actually a one piece dowel crown, then the anticipated cement line *never will be encountered*. When this happens, a decision must be made regarding just how far the dentist is willing to cut axially before concluding that there is no cement line and this is a one-piece casting. This should be judged on the basis of typical preparation design and the restoration's faciolingual dimension. The objective is to cut no deeper than what would normally be considered the typical preparation for that particular situation (Fig. 2-29).

Step 5

Once it is decided that this is not a separate crown and dowel core, the only choice left is to simply prepare the gold as if it were a natural tooth—do axial reduction to accomplish normal retention as well as any other necessary steps in preparing a tooth for a crown. This can be a tedious procedure and somewhat uncomfortable for the patient. However, the only alternative is extraction.

Removal of cast gold inlays

The problem to address when an MOD inlay must be removed from a tooth is inherent in the preparation design. The isthmus is usually narrowest where the triangular ridges approximate each other—midway between the mesial and distal areas of the tooth. Proximal boxes do not present problems since they do not resist displacement of the inlay once the isthmus has been cut through. It is critical to cut the isthmus completely through so that no portion of the dovetail design prevents the two box segments from being moved apart mesially and distally. It is also extremely important here to avoid undue force during removal of the restoration. The preparation design of an MOD inlay is such that by failing to completely cut away the isthmus a minimal force could easily cause the tooth to fracture. Various studies have shown that MOD inlays can predispose the tooth to fracture.[4,5] Therefore, extreme care should be taken to remove all the gold from the isthmus area prior to attempting to remove the rest of the casting from the boxes.

Step 1

Isolate the area with either a rubber dam or a 4 × 4 gauze placed at the back of the oral cavity to prevent aspiration of these small pieces.

Step 2

Using a round-end, cross-cut, nontapered fissure bur such as a no. 1558, cut down through the isthmus, removing the casting all the way to the pulpal floor. Inspect the area of this cut carefully, preferably using magnification to ascertain that no tag of gold connects the two boxes and that no undercut prevents displacement of the resulting casting segments in a proximal direction.

Step 3

Using an instrument such as a large spoon excavator placed into the space between the segments, apply leverage against one of them with the other acting as a fulcrum. Normally, this will cause the cement bond between one of the segments and its box to fail. Before actually removing this segment, turn the spoon around or use the opposite end to apply the same force to the other segment, using the first one as the fulcrum. Even though one of the segments is loose, it can still act as a fulcrum to resist the force, as it is temporarily wedged in between the teeth. When both segments are loosened they can be easily removed with a hemostat or Backhaus clamp.

Step 4

If the spoon excavator does not loosen one part or the other, placing one beak of the Backhaus clamp on the proximal surface of the segment in question and the opposite beak into the cement line between the inlay and pulpal floor will usually release it.

References

1. Oliva, R.A. Review of methods for removing cast gold restorations. J. Am. Dent. Assoc. 99:840–847, 1979.
2. Ishikiriama, A., et al. Temporary cementation of acrylic resin and cast complete crowns. J. Prosthet. Dent. 51:637–641, 1984.
3. Oliva, R.A. Clinical evaluation of a new crown and fixed partial denture remover. J. Prosthet. Dent. 44:267–269, 1980.
4. Fisher, D.W., et al. Photoelastic analysis of inlay and onlay preparations. J. Prosthet. Dent. 33:47–53, 1975.
5. Fisher, D.W., and Caputo, A.A. An analysis of inlay and onlay design using three dimensional photoelasticity. J. Dent. Res. 54(Special Issue A):91, 1975.
6. Mann, A.W., Courtade, G.L., and Sanell, C. The use of pins in restorative dentistry. Part I. Parallel pin retention without using paralleling devices. J. Prosthet. Dent. 15:502–516, 1965.

Additional reading

Abrams, B.L. Simplified removal of defective crowns. Gen. Dent. 26(6):62–64, 1978.

Flashing, D.J. Technique for removal of temporary crowns. Dent. Surv. 48:31, 1972.

Howell, P.G. Assessment of a bur designed for the removal of metal restorations. Br. Dent. J. 21:156–160, 1984.

Kantorowicz, G.F. The repair and removal of bridges. Dent. Pract. Dent. Rec. 21:341–346, 1971.

Karnoff, E.M. Removing cemented crowns and bridges without destroying them. N.Y. J. Dent. 45:158–159, 1975.

Tebrock, O.C. Technique for post-core removal from a crown and a new post-core fabrication. J. Prosthet. Dent. 43:463–466, 1980.

Warren, S.R., and Gutmann, J.L. Simplified method for removing intraradicular posts. J. Prosthet. Dent. 42:353–356, 1979.

Williams, V.D., and Bjorndal, A.M. The Masserann technique for the removal of fractured posts in endodontically treated teeth. J. Prosthet. Dent. 49:46–48, 1983.

Chapter 3

Crown or Pontic Facing Replacement

Every dentist has had a patient present with a bridge or crown with fractured facing or abrasion to the point that it is functionally or esthetically unacceptable. The restoration may have been in the mouth for a short time or for many years. Clinical examination may even reveal good quality margins with no hint of recurrent caries. The restoration could exhibit good contours and occlusion, and radiographs could show no problem. Except for the damaged facing, this restoration is clinically acceptable and shows no evidence of any other defects.

Treatment allows for one of the following alternatives:

1. Leaving the old restoration in place with the defective facing and attendant poor function or esthetics.
2. Removal of the old restoration and fabrication of a new one.
3. Correction of the defect, either by direct or indirect means, without removal of the restoration from the mouth.

Leaving the restoration in place is sometimes an acceptable solution, but often is not. Making a new restoration is the most expensive alternative in terms of time and cost. However, the new restoration may not be as acceptable to the patient as the old one was, if only from a psychological standpoint.

There are limits to these techniques such as the design of the original restoration, as in the following examples:

1. There would be no point in attempting to add any type of material to the defect on the occlusal surface of this porcelain-fused-to-metal (PFM) premolar, since there is insufficient occlusal clearance to begin with (Fig. 3-1).
2. The design of the bridge in this illustration is faulty, and most likely the cause of the failure (Fig. 3-2).
3. In the case of this PFM crown, there is simply no way to gain the needed retention for addition of material without possibly jeopardizing the remaining restoration or the tooth (Fig. 3-3).

There are several methods of correcting the problem while leaving the old restoration in the mouth. It is important to review first the various, sometimes obsolete, methods used to construct these restorations over the past several decades.

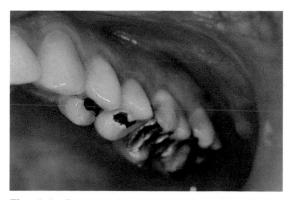

Fig. 3-1 Porcelain-fused-to-metal crown with inadequate occlusal space for porcelain.

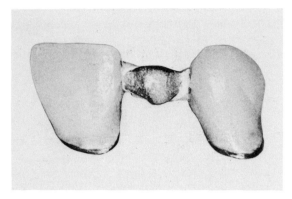

Fig. 3-2 Porcelain-fused-to-metal bridge with improper framework design.

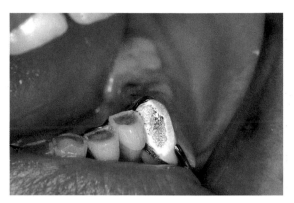

Fig. 3-3 Porcelain-fused-to-metal crown which is not correctable since there is inadequate porcelain for bonding.

Historical perspective

Some of the methods which have been used for developing esthetic facings of crowns or fixed bridges include:

1. Steele's facings
2. Harmony facings
3. Tube pontics
4. Hollenbach facings
5. Various other premade or custom facings

Most of these methods involved a premade porcelain unit cemented onto a casting of some type that was part of the crown or bridge. That the facing was made prior to the casting presents the dentist with having to restore the case using steps in reverse order. A casting in the mouth needing a facing or pontic replaced requires the opposite sequence of the original technique.

Many of these restorations have no other defects outside of the need for facing or pontic replacement. *In keeping with the authors' basic premise guiding all recommendations presented in this work, it is a foregone conclusion that if any of the methods presented are to be used by the dentist, the restorations must be free of any other deficiencies.* The following criteria must be met:

1. All margins must meet the same standard as required when evaluating the crown prior to cementation.
2. Proper contours must be present.
3. The occlusion must be both functional in accordance with the anatomy originally waxed into the restoration, and free of deterioration caused by excessive wear.
4. In the case of a bridge, the hygienic potential should be in evidence. It may be apparent that the patient is not making an adequate attempt to clean the pontic area, but the restoration should at least be free of obviously poor design parameters such as saddle pontic form or inaccessible embrasures.

The dentist should use these techniques for replacement of a facing only if the restoration otherwise meets standard of acceptability. These methods are not put forth as cure-alls for "saving a poor restoration." A defective restoration should be replaced.

Review of facing techniques

Over the years, many different facings have been employed in making fixed bridges and crowns more esthetic. Those of practical interest date from the late 1920s.[1] It was at that time that the first dental castings were made. This introduced the first reasonable method of placing a crown which might need such a facing. These facings generally were cemented to the casting before cementation in the mouth. The method of retention varied, but most shared several common disadvantages:

1. The facing was usually contoured prior to waxing the casting, which made subsequent replacement difficult or impossible.
2. Cement was the primary mechanism for retention. All other retentive features still require cement to ensure success.
3. Porcelain was the most common material for the facing itself, but raised the potential for fracture.
4. Owing to various means for retention of the porcelain to the casting, the facing was prone to fracture because all of these mechanisms tended to weaken the structure of the facing and initiate the propagation of fracture lines.
5. At least on the facings of bridge retainers or single crowns, the facing was dangerously thin.

Most of these problems have been alleviated by the porcelain-fused-to-metal technique. The bond between the fired porcelain and the casting has eliminated the need for any kind of mechanical locks, while reducing the potential for fracture by dispersing stress over the whole bonding area.[2,3]

To understand the obstacles to successfully correcting defects involving these facings, it is important to understand their design and use. This understanding is becoming more significant as the years go by for these reasons:

1. The average dentist today, and certainly the new graduate, will not have had any experience with most of these techniques. He or

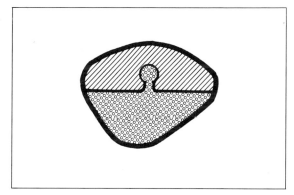

Fig. 3-4 Steele's Trupontic facing showing design of groove in porcelain facing.

she will have been exclusively taught the porcelain-fused-to-metal method.
2. Many restorations placed in the 1950s or 1960s now have defects. Many times patients are seeking some corrective help that would not entail replacing the entire restoration.
3. Financial limitations and the desire of the "insurer" to contain costs through less expensive treatments.

Successfully correcting defects will depend on the dentist's ability, ingenuity, and knowledge of the way the restoration was initially designed and constructed.

Following are some examples of the different methods with which the dentist may be confronted in practice today.

Steele's Trupontic

Steele's Trupontic* was one of the most common methods used prior to porcelain-fused-to-metal in bridge pontics. It consisted of a premade high-fusing porcelain facing available in various forms and shades. The mechanism of retention was tongue and groove, with the groove in the back of the porcelain facing and the tongue in the casting (Fig. 3-4). Hence, a built-in fracture potential existed in the porcelain

*Available through Franklin Dental, Hilgard, Ohio.

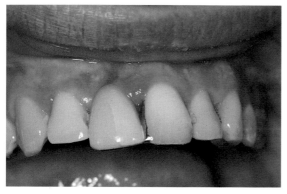

Fig. 3-5 Typical failure of Steele's Trupontic facing, showing fracture line radiating from the groove.

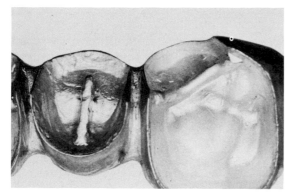

Fig. 3-6a Casting of backing for Steele's Trupontic showing retention ridge.

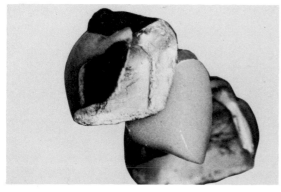

Fig. 3-6b Typical Steele's Trupontic facing as used for a bridge pontic.

facing (Fig. 3-5). The procedure involved selecting the proper facing and grinding it to adapt to the pontic area of the cast so that it satisfied the requirements of the particular dentist or technician for the facial and gingival surfaces of a pontic. At this point, a premade gold backing was trimmed such that when the facing and backing were placed together via the tongue (backing) and the groove (facing), a wax pattern could be completed against the backing that would complete the desired contours for the pontic. The pattern together with the backing was invested, cast, and related to the retainers; the bridge was soldered, and the assembly was checked in the mouth. The final step, just prior to cementation of the bridge, was to cement the facing (Trupontic) to the backing (Figs. 3-6a and b).

This method had all of the general disadvantages listed earlier, plus more:

1. Because the facing was made of a high-fusing porcelain, there were problems related to the coefficient of expansion that made staining and glazing difficult.
2. The intention of the manufacturer was that the facings would be replaceable in the case of a fracture in service, hence the premade gold alloy backing.

If the techniques were done as intended, down to the last detail, this premade backing was the only part of the casting that touched the porcelain facing. However, in practice, this was a very difficult procedure in many cases because the technician had, either inadvertently or by design, actually waxed directly against the facing in some areas. This meant that there would be an interference when attempting to seat a new facing to the existing casting.

Harmony facing

This was also a premade high-fusing porcelain facing, which would be contoured to the residual ridge area of the stone cast, and a backing waxed and cast to fit. Here there was no premade backing.

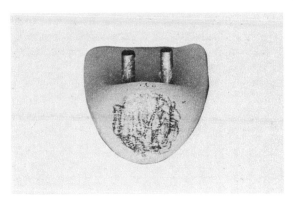

Fig. 3-7 Harmony facing showing pins fused into porcelain at time of manufacture.

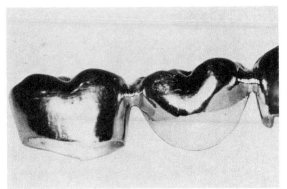

Fig. 3-8a Harmony facing used as a bridge pontic.

The retention consisted of two pins fired into the facing during manufacture. The protruding portions of the pins were cemented into holes created in the casting during the waxup phase. Used primarily as pontics on posterior bridges (Figs. 3-7 and 3-8a and b), Harmony facings have been used for anterior pontics, and are particularly prone to fracture around the pins (Fig. 3-9). One of the most significant differences between the harmony method and the Steele's Trupontics is that the harmony facing had no premade metal backing, which meant that direct replacement was not a possibility. Every backing would be different from all others once the bridge was waxed because each porcelain pontic facing was contoured by a technician as he or she saw fit, before the backing pattern was waxed to it.

The other major difference is in the mechanism for retention, which involved two high-fusing metal (platinum alloy) pins fused to the porcelain facing when manufactured. As with the Trupontic, a built-in fracture potential was thus created, though clinical experience would seem to indicate that it was less problematic.

The primary drawback with this method was probably the difficulty in creating the holes in the cast backing to receive the pins at the time of cementation. Often the procedure was not done as neatly as expected. This resulted in the need for reaming out the holes, which in turn caused

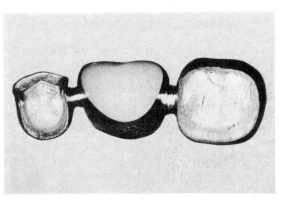

Fig. 3-8b Gingival aspect of a typical-design mandibular Harmony facing bridge pontic.

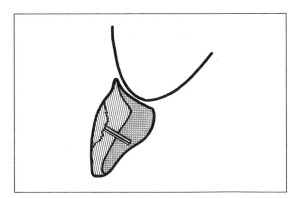

Fig. 3-9 Harmony pontic showing typical fracture radiating from the pins.

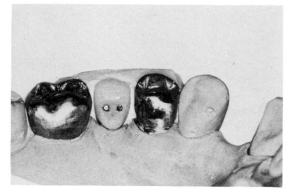

Fig. 3-10a Harmony facing related to bridge retainer castings with backings ready for waxing.

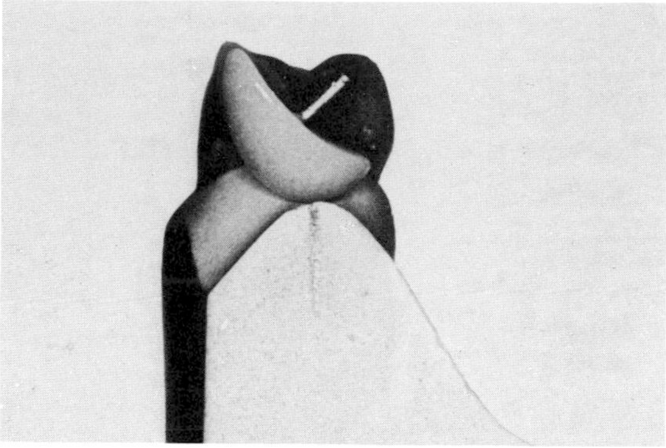

Fig. 3-10b Proximal view of Harmony facing on cast. Pins are in a partially occlusogingival direction.

poor retention. Along with fracture, loss of retention was common. Another serious problem created by the basic design in this technique was the direction of the pins. The pins were directed in an occluso-gingival direction rather than a facio-lingual one (Figs. 3-10a and b). As with the Trupontic, the porcelain facing was normally cemented to the bridge casting prior to cementation of the restoration in the mouth. Although the direction of pin insertion was irrelevant to the porcelain technique, when the casting is in the mouth, the pin direction becomes critical. If the holes are directed toward the ridge, no correction can be successful.

Tube pontic

The tube pontic consisted of a premade porcelain tooth with a hole in the center starting at the gingival aspect. It may or may not have had some kind of separate metal backing, and was always retained by a post fitting into the tube in the porcelain itself (Fig. 3-11). The post was part of the bridge framework and was often seen on removable partial dentures, but could be found on fixed bridges occasionally. It was often done in the mandibular anterior where space for other techniques might be inadequate and where esthetics can be paramount. When these were done in the past as porcelain jacket

crowns, they suffered considerable breakage. Recent attempts to use this method have been more successful, owing to the ability of dentists to use a cast alloy backing onto which porcelain is fired. This is probably the easiest type of pontic to replace in the case of a failure, because the post is visible and accessible.

Hollenbach facing

When the Hollenbach facing was used, a standard denture tooth, rather than one made specifically for such a method, was ground to fit over the facial surface of a preparation. This method is more adaptable to facings on retainers or single crowns than any other method mentioned because no pins are seated into the casting and there are no posts or any other significant retentive features.

The facing was retained by cement and by the minimal "groovelike" retention available at the mesial and distal aspects of the facing area. The wax pattern was adapted to the inside surface of the ground facing, and the crown was cast (Fig. 3-12). In short, the prospect of replacing such a facing simply does not exist. The primary risk when using these facings involved loss or retention and fracture due to very thin ground facing. Space was limited more in the case of a facing on a crown than on a pontic.

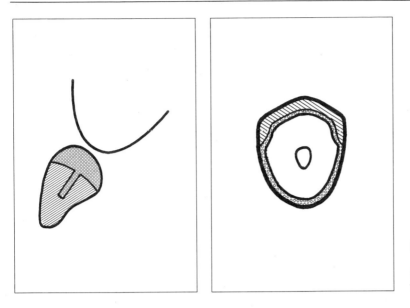

Fig. 3-11 *(far left)* Tube pontic.

Fig. 3-12 *(left)* Hollenbach facing.

These types are difficult and usually impossible to replace in the mouth because of the nearly complete lack of retention form and the fact that the backing was originally waxed to the custom-ground facing.

Methods

The choice of method will depend on several factors. Among these are:

1. The type of facing and backing which were used to construct the original restoration
2. The specific desires of the patient related to such variables as time, esthetic result, and permanence
3. Materials available
4. The dentist's ability and knowledge
5. Forces to be placed on the resulting restoration such as occlusion, with particular emphasis on evaluation of results of long-term wear

The original type of facing will sometimes dictate a straightforward solution, often requiring little more than removal of the remnants of the broken facing prior to replacement. More often it will be necessary to create additional retention by using pin holes, grooves, or roughening the surface, depending on the method of facing replacement.

The importance of the type of backing is from the standpoint of the alloy originally used to cast it. Problems are created by using the newer nonprecious metal alloys. These are much harder and so present difficulties in preparing the needed retentive features.

The desires of the patient must be considered. Some of the methods suggested here, and those which appear in the related literature, are more time-consuming than others. Some are temporary owing either to the material or the method of retention used for that specific technique. In a situation where a correction is being made that is intended to last only until a permanent new restoration can be made, it is not so important to have a long-term success. The esthetics of a finished restoration are less important from a health standpoint, but are often very critical to the patient's feeling of well-being. For example, when one replaces the original high-fusing porcelain facing with a light-cured composite or another resin, less satisfying esthetics can result. This may be acceptable in one patient's situation, but not in another's.

We will attempt to emphasize those features and steps of a given method related directly to the availability and selection of materials and to indicate whether substitution of another material is advisable.

It is in the patient's best interest to be in the care of a dentist who has as many different alternatives as possible for correcting a defect. Otherwise, unless the patient's particular problem happens to fit into that dentist's own limited scope of possibilities, the final result will be a compromise and the patient will not receive the best treatment the profession can offer.

Occlusion is one of the most commonly overlooked considerations in making a treatment decision. It must be appreciated that the occlusion may have undergone major or minor changes since the original restoration. This is particularly true of bruxism where the patient has created large wear facets in the restorations. Bruxism has at least two significant effects on changes related to the facing replacement, which, if disregarded, may bring on the same result as the original facing.

The first is that the original facing may be functioning in a working or balancing position, even if it is not in centric position. This can easily occur from years of wear. It could be said that if the restoration has undergone extreme wear, the entire restoration, rather than just the facing, should be replaced. However, we are referring to cases where the entire mouth has developed a different functional occlusion owing to overall wear. But unless full-mouth reconstruction is being done, the new restoration on which the facing needs to be replaced would need to be designed with the same wear pattern.

Another effect of occlusion is on the casting itself. The backing may have changed shape and thickness and therefore be more likely to deform after the new facing is placed.

If either factor exists, the dentist should seriously consider remaking the restoration, since the chances of successfully satisfying all the criteria for a good fixed prosthodontic restoration are minimal.

Pin-retained porcelain-fused-to-metal replacement facings

This method involves constructing a replacement facing that is retained by pins which are a part of the new casting with a porcelain facing fired onto it similarly to any other porcelain-fused-to-metal restoration. It is primarily used for pontics of fixed bridges, rather than as abutments or single units, because it involves placing two or more pinholes into the metal. While it is sometimes possible to place the necessary retention holes into a crown without jeopardizing either the pulp, if present, or the retention, this is the exception rather than the rule. Basically the procedure consists of making holes in the casting of the bridge, creating an indirect pattern with pins, casting the pattern, then firing with porcelain and cementing.[4]

Method

Step 1

Remove all remnants of the broken facing as well as any areas of the metal casting which would interfere with a facial line of draw. This requires developing retention in a line of draw that is essentially at a right angle to the long axes of the teeth.

Step 2

Plot the placement of the pin holes, then use the flutes on the side of a small round bur, such as a one-quarter or one-half round to make a small dimple at the location of each proposed hole. Generally, two holes are adequate—one toward the mesial aspect and one toward the distal. The importance of the dimples is that by placing these two holes far enough apart for good stability of the replacement casting, they will usually need to be drilled into a surface which is not at a right angle to the drill used for the pinhole itself. The dimples provide a defined starting point for the twist drill used to place the holes (Fig. 3-13).

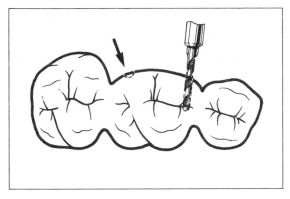

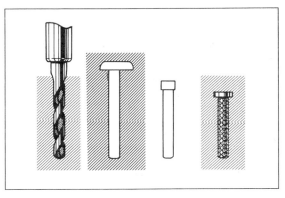

Fig. 3-13 Dimple (as shown by arrow) used for staring hole in pontic casting followed by twist drill to place hole to proper depth.

Fig. 3-14 VIP pin system showing (left to right) twist drill, impression pin with head, pin for temporaries (not used in this method), and iridio-platinum pin for final casting.

Step 3

Drill the pinholes into the metal of the pontic backing to a depth of 2 mm. In the VIP* system of drills and pins, drills of .024 inch are matched with plastic pins of .017 inch and iridio-platinum pins of .007 inch. The system is designed to place pins as part of a casting into dentin. Therefore, there are two types of pins; the plastic pin is used for making the impression, and the iridio-platinum pin is for placing into the wax pattern. The iridio-platinum pin ultimately becomes part of the final restoration after casting (Fig. 3-14).

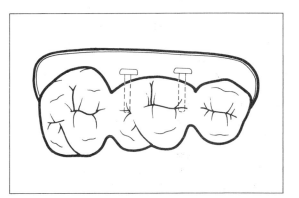

Fig. 3-15 Pontic with holes drilled and impression pins and tray in place.

Step 4

Place impression pins from the VIP kit into the holes to verify their stability. Use an elastomeric impression material in a custom acrylic tray made from the diagnostic cast to make the impression. The tray is made to draw in a facial direction, not in the usual manner—that is, occlusally. It must draw parallel to the direction of the pinholes (Fig. 3-15). The impression should be checked under the microscope for stability and parallelism of the pins.

Step 5

Box the impression and pour it in such a manner as to result in a cast that includes not only the facing area being corrected, but the facial surfaces of the adjacent teeth as well, to aid the technician in contouring the new facing (Fig. 3-16). Note that this type of cast cannot be used for mounting against an opposing cast to articulate the new facial cusp with the existing opposing occlusion. This presents few problems since the facial cusps of the adjacent teeth can be used as guides in building new porcelain with the final adjustment being made in the mouth, prior to glazing the finished porcelain facing.

*Whaledent International, New York, N.Y.

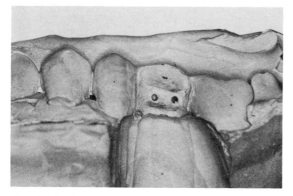

Fig. 3-16 Stone cast showing holes produced by impression pins. Pins have been removed from cast after separation from the impression.

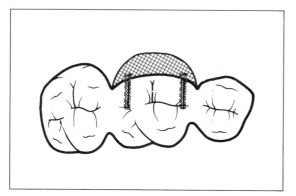

Fig. 3-17 Waxup of full contour of replacement facing on stone cast with iridio-platinum pins in place.

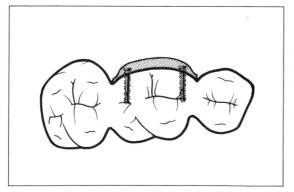

Fig. 3-18 Casting of coping seated on stone cast showing relationship of heads of iridio-platinum pins to casting. Finish lines are visible mesially and distally.

However, if a full-arch cast that can be mounted is necessary, use the following procedure:

1. Make the impression of the facing area as described above, using the impression pins.
2. Leaving that impression in place, make an alginate or hydrocolloid impression over it which reproduces the entire arch.
3. Remove the full-arch impression.
4. Remove the facial impression with pins.
5. Seat the facial impression tray into the corresponding area of the full-arch impression and pour in the normal manner.
6. Separate the two from the cast as in steps 3 and 4.

Step 6

After the cast is separated from the impression, remove the special impression pins from the cast.

Step 7

Place the waxing pins, made of iridio-platinum alloy, into the pinholes in the cast and complete the full-contour waxup (Fig. 3-17). As with any porcelain-fused-to-metal restoration, it is important to complete a full-contour waxup, then to follow with a cutback for the veneering porcelain.

Step 8

Cut back the waxup to provide optimum thickness of porcelain. Normally this will be approximately 1.5 mm, but may vary depending on the requirements of the case (Fig. 3-18).

Finish lines should meet the following requirements:

1. On the mesial and distal surfaces the finish lines should take the form of a chamfer approximately 1/2 to 1 mm deep.
2. On the gingival surface, the finish line should be essentially a very shallow chamfer, with the junction between the replacement backing and the existing restoration just facial to

the area of closest approximation to the ridge.

3. On the occlusal or incisal, the finish line will usually be a simple 90° butt joint.

Step 9

Withdraw the waxup from the cast, after attaching a sprue in the center of the facial surface, with auxiliary sprues added as needed, depending on the type of alloy to be used for the casting. Make the casting and remove the sprues.

Step 10

Verify the casting fit on the stone cast, and in the mouth, if desired. Generally, it is not necessary to have a separate try-in in the mouth, and it is more efficient to wait until the porcelain is fired onto the casting. Trying-in the casting prior to porcelain addition, if a full-arch cast for occlusion was not used, affords an opportunity to make exact determination of the ideal contour of the occlusal or incisal edge of the new facing. The following technique is often helpful:

1. Add wax to the porcelain veneering area in the laboratory and carve to the anticipated contour, paying particular attention to length as related to the eccentric occlusal positions.
2. Place the casting with the trial waxup of the porcelain veneer in the mouth and instruct the patient to move to the appropriate functional positions.
3. Make any indicated adjustments and check the occlusion again.
4. Make an impression for a cameo cast of the facial surfaces of the trial wax-up and the adjacent teeth with alginate in a standard quadrant tray.
5. Pour this impression and use the resulting cast while baking the porcelain.

The extra effort and chair time is justified only in certain unusual cases, such as severe wear, where the eccentric occlusion is of primary importance.

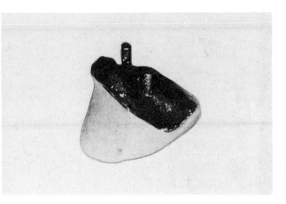

Fig. 3-19 Finished casting with baked porcelain facing.

Step 11

The porcelain is baked, contoured, and either glazed or returned for try-in unglazed (Fig. 3-19). Try the final replacement facing in the mouth. Verify, adjust, stain, and glaze as indicated. If each step in the procedure has been carefully followed, some of these additional steps may be unnecessary.

Step 12

Cement the replacement facing with a zinc-phosphate cement, paying particular attention to getting cement into the pinholes. Retention for this method depends on the pins being cemented adequately into the holes in the existing bridge casting. As with any pin-retained casting, the cement at the interface between the two gold castings affords no usable retention. Instead, the entire retention comes from the cement around the pins in their holes.

Variations for thin backings

Occasionally, in anterior bridge pontics the dentist will find that the metal backing is too thin to provide a pinhole deep enough for adequate retention provided for in the previous technique (Fig. 3-20). When the criterion of 2 mm deep holes cannot be met, employ the following procedure:

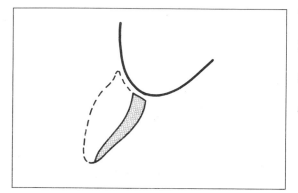

Fig. 3-20 Problem presented by a thin backing on anterior bridge pontic.

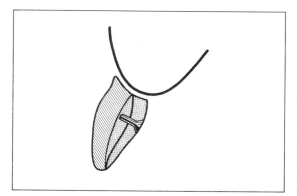

Fig. 3-21 Final result in the case of thin backing with pinholes drilled completely through and countersunk on the lingual aspect.

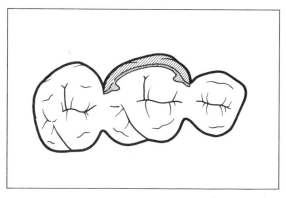

Fig. 3-22 Replacement facing design using mesial and distal grooves instead of pins for retention of replacement facing on either a crown or a pontic.

1. Plot the pinholes as described in the previous section.
2. Drill the holes all the way through the backing so that they exit on the lingual surface.
3. Countersink the holes on the lingual surface with a no. 6 round bur.
4. Make the pins of an alloy softer than those in the VIP kit so they can be burnished. To do this, use an appropriate size of nylon or plastic pins, so that after burnout and casting all pins will be made of the same alloy as the parent casting.
5. Follow the previous technique up to cementation. Upon cementation, the pins protruding past the lingual surface are finished off and burnished flush with the surface, locking them into the countersink (Fig. 3-21).

Groove-retained porcelain-fused-to-metal replacement facings

The groove-retention method is similar in many respects to the pin-retention method. After the backing has been constructed and is ready to receive porcelain, the methods are essentially the same.

Retention is provided by two grooves, one each at the mesial and distal extremes of the facing area (Fig. 3-22). An adequate bulk of metal is required in the existing bridge pontic to allow placement of two grooves that will resist displacement in a facial direction. There must be enough length, at least 3 mm in most cases, to attain adequate retention with no tendency toward dislodgement in an occlusal direction.

This method is more applicable to pontics than to bridge retainers or single crowns because of the limited thickness of metal in those units.

Method

Step 1

Remove all remaining porcelain from the area to be corrected, leaving only the metal surface of the existing restoration on the unit to be corrected. It is good practice to make an alginate impression of the remaining restoration and pour it in a fast-setting plaster. The resulting cast should then be scrutinized to make judgments in several areas which will have a bearing on the procedure to be followed:

Examine the space available for construction of the new facing, including the metal backing, and the thickness of porcelain, which affects esthetics. Bear in mind that one reason for breakage of the original facing might have been that it was too thin. If so, you will need to accomplish a greater reduction than originally provided in the bridge framework.

The potential for developing a proper line of draw for the new backing must be considered in relation not only to the adjacent units, but also to the ridge (Fig. 3-23). Often, if a porcelain-fused-to-metal restoration is involved, the cutback for the porcelain veneer may have been done such as to continue in a curve from the facial onto the gingival aspect of the pontic casting (Fig. 3-24). In this case the line of draw as indicated by the arrow would result in an undercut in the region circled at the gingival aspect of the pontic. This problem is compounded in a pontic design that involves veneering the entire gingival surface of the pontic with porcelain instead of metal in contact with the tissue. In the latter situation it is unlikely that the technique described will be usable; the restoration will usually need to be remade. However, if the curve and resulting undercut are small, one of two courses should be followed:

1. Modify the line of draw on the preparation to be accomplished such that the grooves are farther facially at the occlusal aspect than at the gingival (Fig. 3-25).
2. Use the previously described pin-retained method. In this manner, the line of draw can

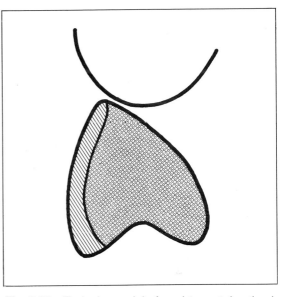

Fig. 3-23 Typical porcelain-fused-to-metal cutback on a maxillary pontic, showing minimal undercut near the gingival aspect.

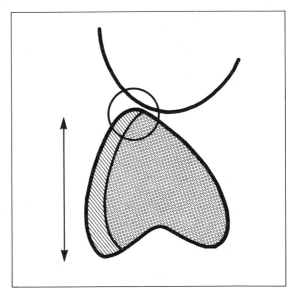

Fig. 3-24 Problem created when the original porcelain-fused-to-metal cutback results in a significant undercut at the gingival aspect *(circle)*.

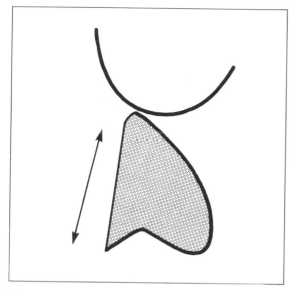

Fig. 3-25 Modification in line of draw helping to eliminate the undercut.

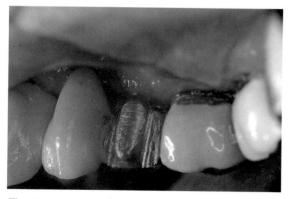

Fig. 3-26 Facing replacement preparation on a pontic with grooves cut on the mesial and distal aspects of the facial surface.

be developed in a facio-lingual direction, thus eliminating the problem presented at the gingival aspect of the pontic.

Since the subtle curvature is frequently difficult to see in the mouth, determining the presence or absence of this often overlooked contour problem is one of the major values of the cast.

Step 2

Using a 12-fluted finishing bur with straight sides, smooth the entire surface of the existing pontic casting to eliminate any undercuts to the chosen line of draw. This can be done effectively by painting the surface with a mixture of rouge and chloroform, allowing it to dry, and running the bur over the surface. The low spots will be indicated by areas of rouge left in the depressions. Smoothing should continue until all surface roughness is gone (Fig. 3-26).

Step 3

Utilizing a no. 700 or no. 701 nondentate carbide-tapered fissure bur, place two grooves in the line of draw you have selected. One groove will be placed at the mesial and one at the distal aspect of the facing area of the existing casting. The grooves must draw both in relation to each other and in relation to the adjacent units of the bridge. This line of draw usually will be parallel to the long axis of the teeth in the quadrant, but will often need modification, as mentioned in Step 1. Axially these grooves should be approximately 0.5 to 1 mm deep.

Create a definite seat of some type to limit the travel of the replacement facing gingivally upon seating. This can be accomplished in one of two ways: The grooves should have a very definite gingival seat (Fig. 3-27), or a distinct bevel can be placed on the occlusal surface of the remaining bridge casting such that even though the grooves themselves have no seat, due to lack of space, the movement of the replacement facing gingivally is stopped as the new casting is seated onto the bevel (Fig. 3-28).

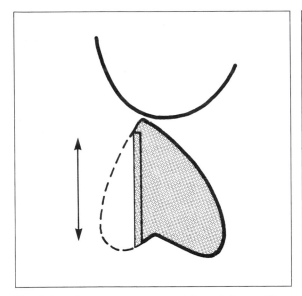

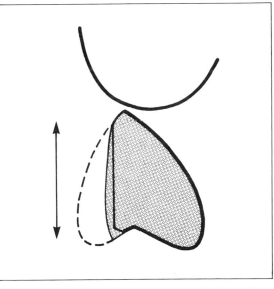

Fig. 3-27 Groove cut in correct line of draw with a definite gingival stop.

Fig. 3-28 Groove cut in correct line of draw with a bevel on the occlusal aspect.

Step 4

Make an impression of the quadrant using any standard impression technique. A simple and convenient method in this instance is the Coe Check-Bite Tray* described in chapter 9. This impression system is particularly good for this application, since no removable die need be generated, and time is saved by obtaining both the maxillary and mandibular impressions concurrently. In the interest of accuracy, carefully remove the impression along the line of draw of the two grooves. Any severe undercuts or malposed teeth interfering with this line of withdrawal of the impression should be blocked out with a soft wax prior to making the impression.

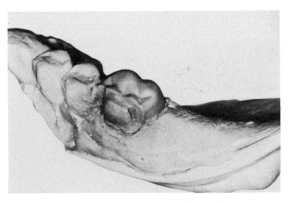

Fig. 3-29 Stone cast of a preparation using grooves on the mesial and distal aspects of the facial surface of a bridge retainer.

Step 5

Pour the impression such as to generate mounted maxillary and mandibular casts in a densite stone. Usually, an individual cast of the involved quadrant will be adequate (Fig. 3-29).

*Coe Laboratories, Inc., Chicago, Ill.

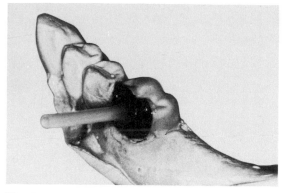

Fig. 3-30 Wax pattern on cast with cutback done, and sprue attached.

Step 6

The pattern for the metal backing is waxed on the cast, with no other preparation of the stone cast needed (Fig. 3-30). The following goals should be kept in mind while doing this wax pattern:

1. Perfectly reproduced grooves to prevent decreased retention
2. Backing that allows for the proper thickness of porcelain for optimal esthetics
3. Well-defined featheredge finish lines, lingual to the grooves, at the mesial and distal aspects, so that when the replacement facing is

seated, metal rather than porcelain contacts the existing restoration.

Cast the backing in the usual manner.

Step 7

Remove the sprue and prepare the surface to receive porcelain. The backing should be tried onto the stone cast to verify fit (Figs. 3-31a and b). As with all castings, this one should be inspected under the microscope prior to trying it onto the stone cast. Remove all blebs.

Step 8

Bake the porcelain onto the facing using the facial contour of the adjacent teeth as a guide (Fig. 3-32).

Step 9

Try the resulting replacement facing in the mouth. Check the occlusion in working position, adjust shade and contour as with any porcelain-fused-to-metal restoration, and cement it with a zinc-phosphate cement (Fig. 3-33).

This procedure is most applicable for pontics, where there is greater space for the grooves, which allows for greater safety (Figs. 3-34a to d).

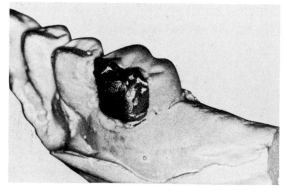

Fig. 3-31a Casting ready for porcelain.

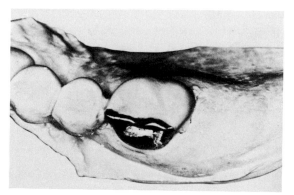

Fig. 3-31b Casting ready for porcelain showing small collar occlusally.

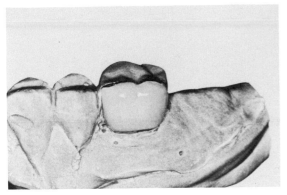

Fig. 3-32 Completed replacement facing on stone cast.

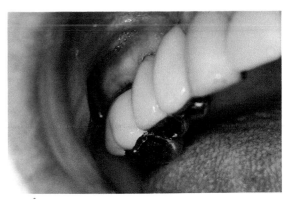

Fig. 3-33 Replacement facing cemented in mouth.

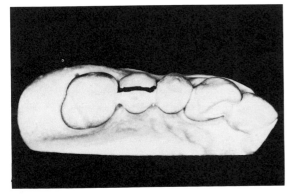

Fig. 3-34a Replacement facing using grooves to replace a lost facing on a bridge pontic.

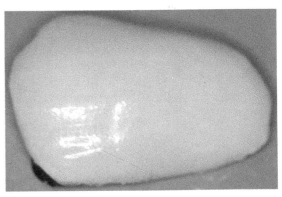

Fig. 3-34b Completed facing.

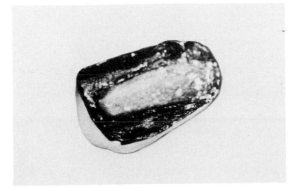

Fig. 3-34c Inside surface of completed facing showing grooves, usually more retentive than is possible on a retainer.

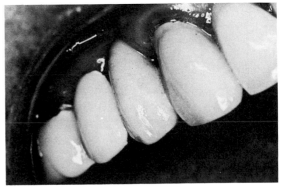

Fig. 3-34d Completed facing in mouth.

Replacement of Steele's Trupontic with plastic

The following methods can be used to correct a Steele's Trupontic that has succumbed to its built-in fracture potential:

1. Replacement with a new porcelain facing from the manufacturer was the basic method intended when the facings were first designed. In actual practice, however, this is usually unsuccessful because parts of the casting often interfere with the seating of a new prefabricated facing. Also, facings of this type are not readily available today.
2. Replacement with a prefabricated facing made of plastic, a material less likely to become a victim of the same fate. Again, fit is difficult in many cases.
3. Replacement with a custom-made plastic facing, designed to fit that particular backing. This is the method to be described here, and is applicable in most cases.

Method

Step 1

Remove any remnants of cement or old porcelain facing material from the original backing.

Step 2

Make an impression of the area of the bridge. This impression must include the remainder of the bridge itself, and any adjacent teeth that will help development of proper contour.

Step 3

In most cases, it will be necessary to make an impression of the opposing arch for purposes of occlusion. Pour the casts in a densite stone (Fig. 3-35).

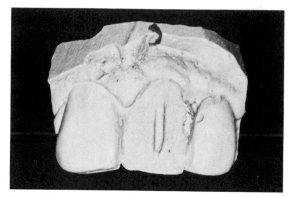

Fig. 3-35 Stone cast of backing after loss of a Steele's facing showing retentive ridge.

Step 4

Mount the casts as indicated in the particular case.

Step 5

Develop the actual replacement facing in either of two ways:

1. Light-cured composite resin. Lubricate the stone cast of the backing with a separating medium such as Alcote.* The appropriate shade of the composite material of choice is adapted onto the model, shaped to the desired contour and then cured with the proper light source. Often it will be wise to use the opaque material for the particular system being used, since in this case, the material will be placed on top of a gold casting rather than on tooth structure. Since this is not actually to be a bonded composite restoration, it is not necessary to use the unfilled resin under the composite as would normally be done.

2. Conventional acrylic resin. Lubricate the stone cast of the backing with a separating medium, in this case a standard die lubricant such as Die Lube.** Develop a wax pattern of the proper contour, and invest it similarly as for

*L. D. Caulk Co., Milford, Del.
**J. M. Ney Co., Bloomfield, Conn.

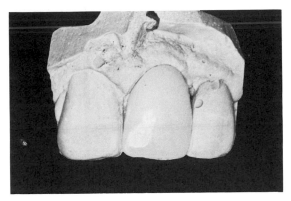

Fig. 3-36 Replacement acrylic facing ready for use.

the heat curing of acrylic facings on cast gold bridges. The stone cast (instead of the bridge casting) is invested in the lower half of a small flask, and the facial surface of the facing itself is invested in the upper half of the flask. The wax is flushed out and replaced by the acrylic resin, which is then heat-cured.

Step 6

In either case, finish, polish, and stain the facing (Fig. 3-36).

Step 7

Cement the facing to the bridge backing in the patient's mouth using a standard zinc-phosphate cement.

Pontic or facing replacement using bonding techniques

With the increased use of porcelain-fused-to-metal crowns and bridges in recent years, dentists are seeing fractured porcelain facings more often. When the defect is small or located where it does not detract esthetically, the dentist may sometimes smooth the edges and leave the defect. This correction is simple, inexpensive, and acceptable. However, frequently the

fracture is so large or so unesthetic that more definitive treatment is required. Often, the best treatment is to replace the entire restoration, while at other times it is desirable and acceptable to correct the defect in a more conservative manner.

When the original porcelain-fused-to-metal restoration was fabricated in the laboratory, the porcelain was baked onto the metal at a high temperature and an intermolecular bond was formed between the metal and the porcelain.[5] It is rarely possible to rebake porcelain once the appliance has been cemented in the mouth, as this would require removal of the casting from the tooth without any damage occurring to either, a highly unusual situation.

The correction described here applies only where the fracture line passes through the porcelain, not where there are large areas of metal exposed (Fig. 3-37). The bonding procedures described rely on fusion between the added material and the old porcelain, not directly to the metal. It is assumed that if the bond between metal and porcelain is adequate to withstand the force that resulted in the fracture of the porcelain, it is still strong enough to act as the retention between metal and porcelain. Mechanical retention can be obtained where there is insufficient area of porcelain for bonding, that is, where the majority of the exposed surface

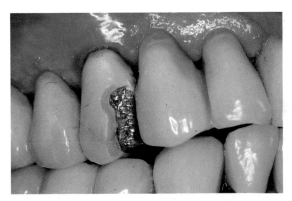

Fig. 3-37 Fractured porcelain-fused-to-metal facing that is not likely to be successfully corrected because most of the area is exposed metal—there is little porcelain with which to bond.

after the failure is metal. These may involve grooves, roughening, and so forth, but whatever method is used, it is important to realize that it is mechanical retention, which is probably not as strong as the original intermolecular bond.

Several bonding agents for porcelain corrections in the mouth have been introduced in recent years.[6–11] Some manufacturers have made claims about their product implying that the material is capable of correcting any defect. There is little research to support such claims, but so far, clinical experience would seem to predict a rather high level of success for many of these products. The area recommended by the authors at this time is bonding of composite resins to the remaining porcelain after a fracture of some of the material. Bonding to exposed metal is less researched and will require more work before it can be handled as routinely as bonding to porcelain.

The use of silane solutions as a porcelain bonding (surface preparation) agent has been known since the early 1960s. Studies have shown that silane can be used to bond porcelain to various materials, primarily composite resins.[12] In the following section we will present a technique, with variations, which can be effective in many cases for correcting defects in porcelain in the patient's mouth. There are currently several "porcelain repair systems" on the market. Most of them rely on a silane solution to prepare the surface of the porcelain to receive a composite repair material. It is important to follow the manufacturer's instructions to achieve the greatest degree of success, although it may be necessary to modify the technique for a given situation based on sound restorative principles. Note that research continues in this area, and that new materials and techniques are frequently advocated. The dentist must carefully evaluate any claims to determine which products are effective.

It is important to be aware of the limits of this technique. For example, the larger the fracture or the more metal that is exposed, the less likely is success. Also, areas of the mouth exposed to heavy occlusion or excessive forces tend to be less successful. Conversely, when the defect is small with little or no metal exposed, or in areas which are out of occlusion, this method can be very reliable. However, similar situations in different patients can often have different results, and what did not work with one patient may be successful with another. After making an accurate assessment of the situation it is incumbent upon the dentist to indicate to the patient that success cannot be insured and that the restoration may still need replacement.

Method

Step 1

Check occlusion to determine the limits to rebuilding the fractured porcelain to the desired contour. Pay attention to any excursive movements that can shear off the new material, particularly at incisal or occlusal angles. If an interference caused the initial fracture, it is unlikely that subsequent treatment will succeed if the cause of the original failure is not first eliminated. It is unwise to rebuild the former contour if that will result in application of the same forces to the correction as those applied to the original porcelain. However, it may be easy to make the correction with the new material and simultaneously eliminate the adverse vector of force by making an acceptable esthetic compromise. A trial waxup in the mouth is advisable in order to see what actually can be done and thereby avoid needless difficulty in the future.

Step 2

Mix silane solution according to directions. Prepare the material as indicated while the next several steps are taken, and the solution will be ready when needed. In the Vivadent* system, this preparation of individual batches of the bonding agent is essential. Note that the prepared material must be used within 24 hours. In the Kerr** system, there are separate etchant

*Vivadent (USA) Inc., Tonawanda, N.Y.
**Kerr/Sybron Manufacturing Co., Romulus, Mich.

and bonding liquids, such that it is not necessary to prepare the material ahead of time. It is important to follow the manufacturer's directions for the specific system being used.

Step 3

Select the proper shade of any light-cured composite to match the remaining porcelain by using the appropriate shade guide for the material. Have more than one composite system available to increase the range of shade selections. The problem of attaining an acceptable esthetic result is compounded by the ever-increasing number of different porcelain systems being developed, many of which use principles of manufacture unfamiliar to the average practitioner.[13]

Modern composites are generally shaded to be esthetically satisfying when they are in contact with natural tooth enamel instead of porcelain. The dentist working with composites and porcelains must arrive at the correct shade through experimentation, using natural or color-corrected light sources.

A light-cured composite offers several advantages over conventional composites. Among them are:

1. Increased working time to allow more exacting placement of material
2. Superior color stability over conventional composite resins
3. Generally a higher degree of polishability due to smaller particle sizes

Most curing lights on the market will cure any composite at depths of 1 to 3 mm. To ascertain whether a particular light will cure a specific composite, place a small amount of material on a pad of paper, cure it, then section the composite to check the depth of the cure.

Step 4

Applying a rubber dam is less critical than when bonding to natural teeth, but it can be very helpful in making these corrections. It will help

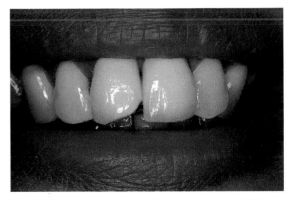

Fig. 3-38 Porcelain-fused-to-metal crown with incisal fracture.

to avoid contamination of the porcelain surface and increase visibility, particularly in relation to adjacent teeth and their respective contours.

Step 5

Smooth down any rough or unsupported porcelain with a white stone. Remove the glaze on the remaining porcelain adjacent to the fracture (Fig. 3-38). If the glaze is not removed, the retention of the composite is severely reduced and failures are more likely.[10] This is done by bevelling the porcelain for at least 1 mm around the fractured area. This bevel also provides a larger area of porcelain to which the composite will adhere. It may be necessary to bevel a larger area, particularly if a significant amount of metal is exposed, reducing the area available for bonding to old porcelain.

Step 6

Add mechanical retention whenever possible to do so without damaging the metal or remaining porcelain. This can be accomplished by one of the following:

1. Roughen exposed metal with a coarse diamond stone. Run the stone in two directions at right angles to one another to produce a grid of scratches for better retention.

73

2. Place retention grooves in sharp internal line angles where an adequate thickness of metal exists. This will also provide significant retention if it can be accomplished without perforating the metal. This last danger, obviously, can limit greatly the usefulness of this particular step.

3. Occasionally, when a previous correction has failed and remaking the restoration is the only choice, placing undercuts in the porcelain, in combination with the silane, may provide sufficient retention of the new material. However, it must be emphasized that placement of any undercuts in the porcelain clearly violates the principles of maintaining strength in the porcelain restorations and increases the risk for failure of the remaining facing. This method should only be used as a last resort, and the risks of further failure should be made very clear to the patient.

Step 7

Clean the entire surface of the porcelain and metal, if any is exposed, with pumice, and rinse with water. Dry with air. A paste containing fluoride should not be used, as it will be detrimental to the development of a good bond.

Step 8

Clean the surface with orthophosphoric acid and rinse with water thoroughly. Dry with clean, oil-free air, using a bulb syringe, rather than the one on the dental unit. It is essential from this step on to keep the area free of contaminants such as saliva until the new composite material has been cured.

Step 9

Mask any exposed metal by mixing the opaquing powder and liquid to a thin creamy mix and applying a thin layer. Let it dry. An additional layer may be necessary to completely cover the metal. It is necessary to work quickly, since the liquid evaporates rapidly. Care should be taken to see that no excess is placed on the remaining porcelain, since this procedure only masks out the color of the material under it, and there is no bond involved. This step accomplishes the same end as an opaque porcelain layer in a porcelain-fused-to-metal restoration. A useful variation has been described by Barreto and Bottaro.[12]

Step 10

Using a disposable brush or a cotton pellet, place freshly prepared silane solution on the porcelain area to be bonded to, and leave there for 3 minutes. Allow to dry or use a light stream of air 6 to 8 inches from the tooth. As previously mentioned, this air should be free of oil, which would likely decrease the dependability of the bond.

Step 11

Place a thin layer of an unfilled light-cured resin of the operator's choice and cure with the appropriate light according to the manufacturer's directions. Add the filled resin and form to the desired contour and again cure with the light. If necessary, more material may be added as long as the surface has not been contaminated.

Step 12

Remove excess and do gross shaping with composite finishing burs, as one would with any composite restoration.

Step 13

Carefully check the occlusion, after removing the rubber dam if one was used, to be sure the restoration is not high in centric or any other excursions. Any interferences can cause failure in a short time.

Step 14

Polish, using the various grades of finishing discs that are a part of the normal regimen for composite restorations (Fig. 3-39).

This method can be used to perform satisfactory corrections in cases where a great amount of metal is exposed, providing that there is adequate procelain surrounding it for good silanizing and, therefore, a good quality bond.

Correction of damaged acrylic veneer

Acrylic veneers have been used for many years as facings for crowns and bridges. With the increase of porcelain-to-metal restorations, they are now used less frequently. However, there are many in the mouth which have been in place for several years and some dentists still use this restoration. As long as this technique is used, the dentist should know how to rectify the failures without necessarily redoing the whole restoration. Drawbacks of acrylic are the susceptibility to abrasion and discoloration (Fig. 3-40). As it gets thinner, it becomes increasingly unesthetic.

A patient may present with an acrylic-to-metal restoration which is clinically acceptable except for a worn or missing facing. Occlusion, margins, contacts, and contours are all satisfactory but the appearance is poor owing to a thin, discolored, or missing facing. When initially completed, this type of restoration relies solely upon mechanical retention of one form or another to retain the facing. Zephre loops as well as small buttons and undercuts in other areas are common forms of retention (Fig. 3-41). Since failure of the facing is usually due to abrasion of the acrylic, the retention is often still present and can be used for intraoral refurbishing.

Use of cold-cure acrylic to replace the missing facing is simple but cannot be used over the long term owing to rapid discoloration. A much longer lasting solution is the use of light-cured composites utilizing the original mechanical retention. Light-cured composites are preferable to conventional composites because of ease of handling, increased working time, and superior color stability. The following technique involves

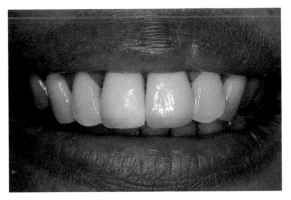

Fig. 3-39 Completed bonded composite resin correction.

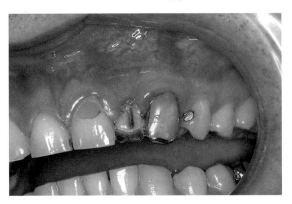

Fig. 3-40 Older unfilled plastic facing showing typical wear and discoloration.

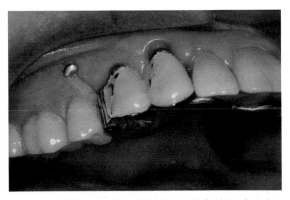

Fig. 3-41 Worn older unfilled plastic facing showing retentive loops.

replacing acrylic facings when no acrylic remains. A method for handling worn facings or cases where some of the facing remains will be discussed later.

Method: No remaining acrylic

Step 1

Thoroughly check the occlusion to determine what limitations there may be. Careful attention must be paid to any excursive movements that can shear off any replacement, particularly when the site is an anterior incisal angle. If interferences were the cause of the initial failure, they must be corrected prior to rebuilding the facing, though most failures are caused by abrasion.

Step 2

Select the proper shade of light-cured composite using the shade guide for the material to be used. Have more than one composite system available to increase the selection of shades.

Step 3

Verify that the remaining retention on the metal is as retentive as possible since this will hold the restoration in place. If the retention is in the form of undercuts around the outside, the internal angles should be accentuated if this can be done without causing perforations. If retention is by means of loops or beads protruding from the metal, they should be free of remaining acrylic. Any small islands of acrylic left on the metal should also be removed.

Step 4

Roughen remaining metal surface. Grooves placed in the metal surface with a coarse diamond will add to the retention. These grooves should be placed in two separate directions at right angles to each other, leaving a cross-grid,

which will aid retention. Care must be taken so that no retentive beads are dislodged. Apply rubber dam, though this step will be optional, and clean area with a pumice solution, wash, rinse, and dry it.

Step 5

Mask the exposed metal by covering it with the opaque material available in the various porcelain repair systems to prevent the color of the metal from showing. Mix opaque powder and liquid monomer to a thin creamy consistency, and quickly apply a thin layer to the metal, noting that more than one layer may be needed. Care should be taken to keep retention areas free of this opaque material, but if it gets into the retention areas, clean the areas with a hand instrument. External margins should also be kept free of the opaque material.

Step 6

Place unfilled resin, ensuring that it engages whatever mechanical retention is available. Place a thin layer of unfilled resin over the entire area to be restored, and cure it with visible light according to manufacturer's directions.

Step 7

Place filled resin. Composite filling material of the proper shade should be placed over the entire area to be restored. Shape and contour with slight excess and then cure with visible light. If undercontoured areas exist, add more material and cure it if it has not been contaminated. If it has been contaminated with saliva, it will be necessary to clean it with pumice and thoroughly rinse and dry before adding more material. This may be necessary if the rubber dam was not used.

Step 8

Reduce excess composite and proceed with gross shaping with a green or white stone, and remove the rubber dam.

Step 9

Carefully check the occlusion to ensure the restoration is not high in centric, or in any excursions. Adjust as necessary, smooth, and polish as with any composite using progressively finer stones, discs, and finishing strips.

This technique provides a method of restoring acrylic facings on crowns and bridges which have been lost. With minimum time and expense, the patient will have a lasting restoration.

Method: Some acrylic remaining

One of the objectives of the previous method is to remove old acrylic from the crown without damaging the retention. As long as the original retentive features are present, adding composite as a facing is very predictable and reliable. However, when a significant layer of acrylic must be removed, the dentist runs the risk of simultaneously removing the retentive features. This is especially true where the retention was achieved by use of beads protruding from the surface of the casting facing.

Adding a composite material to an existing acrylic facing is often workable, although the quality of the fusion is questionable because of years of contamination of the old material. The advantage is that the remaining old acrylic is well-retained while the rest of the facing has been lost which indicates that retention is satisfactory and if the new material fuses adequately, the correction may be successful for a fairly long time.

Step 1

Carefully check the occlusion to determine if there are problems related to functional movements of the teeth in the facing area which might cause failure again. Remove as much of the old acrylic facing as possible without destroying the retention. A fresh area of acrylic needs to be exposed all over the surface for the best possible bonding. Use a coarse diamond in order to leave minute grooves in the acrylic which will enhance retention. The grooves should be placed at approximately right angles to each other. This is the weak link in this procedure because the acrylic has absorbed the intraoral fluids over years and may prevent adequate bonding. Use the diamond to roughen any exposed metal.

Step 2

Select the appropriate shade of the light-cured composite resin. It is advisable to have as many different types of this material available as possible, since we are not using it against natural tooth structure the way the manufacturer intended.

Step 3

Accentuate the retention when possible, and bear in mind that the old acrylic is retained by either beads or loops placed when the crown was cast. The new material must be retained by other means, and mere reliance on the adhesion to the old material is risky. Other mechanical retention should be developed where possible, and the patient should be prepared for the restoration to be remade if *necessary*, because the dentist cannot ensure that this procedure will be successful.

Step 4

Place the rubber dam, and clean the facing area with a prophy cup or brush, and pumice. Rinse completely, and place orthophosphoric acid. Rinse the entire area thoroughly for at least 30 seconds, then dry completely. This step is essential for increasing the chances for success of the correction.

Step 5

Mask any exposed metal, except retentive areas, with the opaque material that can be found in porcelain repair kits on the market. Place a thin layer of an unfilled light-cured resin, and cure with the appropriate light according to the manufacturer's directions. Add the filled resin, form to the desired contour, and cure with the light. Add more material if necessary, as long as the surface has not been contaminated.

Step 6

Remove excess and do gross shaping with green or white stones or composite finishing burs as with any composite restoration. Carefully check the occlusion, after removing the rubber dam if one was used, and ensure that the restoration is not high in centric or in excursions because any interference can rapidly cause failure. Use the various grades of finishing discs to polish.

References

1. Tylman, S.D., and Tylman, S.G. Theory and Practice of Crown and Bridge Prosthodontics. 4th ed. St. Louis: The C.V. Mosby Co., 1960.
2. Yamada, H. (ed.) Dental Porcelain—The State of the Art. Los Angeles: University of Southern California Press, 1977.
3. Tuccillo, J.J., and Cascone, P.J. The evolution of porcelain-fused-to-metal (PFM) alloy system. *In* McLean, J.W. (ed.) Dental Ceramics: Proceedings of the First International Symposium on Ceramics. Chicago: Quintessence Publ. Co., 1983.
4. Mann, A.W., et al. The use of pins in restorative dentistry. J. Prosthet. Dent. 15:502–515, 1965.
5. McLean, J.W. The Science and Art of Dental Ceramics. Chicago: Quintessence Publ. Co., 1980.
6. Nowlin, T.P., et al. Evaluation of the bonding of three porcelain repair systems. J. Prosthet. Dent. 46:516–518, 1981.
7. Highton, R.M., et al. Effectiveness of porcelain repair systems. J. Prosthet. Dent. 42:292–294, 1979.
8. Eames, W.B., and Rogers, L.B. Porcelain repairs: Retention after one year. Operative Dent. 4:75–77, 1979.
9. Eames, W.B., et al. Bonding agents for repairing porcelain and gold: An evaluation. Operative Dent. 2:118–124, 1977.
10. Newburg, R., and Pameijer, C.H. Composite resins bonded to porcelain with silane solution. J. Am. Dent. Assoc. 96:288–291, 1978.
11. Myerson, R.L. Effects of silane bonding of acrylic resins to porcelain on porcelain structure. J. Am. Dent. Assoc. 78:113–119, 1969.
12. Barreto, M.T., and Bottaro, B.F. A practical approach to porcelain repair. J. Prosthet. Dent. 48:349–351, 1982.
13. Preston, J.D. Current status of shade selection and color matching. Quint. Int. 16:47–58, 1985.

Additional reading

Aaronson, S. Addition of a pontic to a preexisting fixed bridge. Dent. Surv. 54:40–41, 1978.
Anusavice, K.J. Identification of fracture zones in PFM by ESCA analysis. J. Prosthet. Dent. 42:417–421, 1979.
Aspes, T., and McIlwain, J.E., Jr. Restorative technic to repair pontics. Dent. Surv. 49:24, 1973.
Bakland, L.K. Replacing porcelain veneers in the mouth. Quint. Int. 3:45–49, 1972.
Bruggers, H. Repair technique for fractured anterior facings. J. Am. Dent. Assoc. 98:947–948, 1979.
Cavel, W.T., et al. The replacement of abraded full crown facings with acrylic veneer facings. Quint. Int. 13:847–849, 1982.
Dent, R.J. Repair of porcelain fused to metal restorations. J. Prosthet. Dent. 41:661–664, 1979.
Dragan, W.B. Esthetic replacement of acrylic veneers on permanently cemented crowns and fixed partial dentures. Quint. Int. 3:53–60, 1972.
Eckstein, E.C. Replacement of acrylic facings on a fixed partial prosthesis. J. Bergen City Dent. Soc. 44:20–21, 1978.
Eisenbrand, G.F. Simplified composite technic for placing porcelain pontics. Dent. Surv. 51:34–35, 1975.
Ferrando, J.P., et al. Tensile strength and microleakage of porcelain repair materials. J. Prosthet. Dent. 50:44–50, 1983.
Jochen, D.G. Composite resin repair of porcelain denture teeth. J. Prosthet. Dent. 38:673–679, 1977.
Johnson, E.P. Saving a bridge. Dent. Surv. 55:44, 1979.
Rehany, A., and Stern, N. A method of refacing cemented veneered crowns. J. Prosthet. Dent. 38:158–160, 1977.
Rehany, A., et al. Repair of fractured porcelain jacket crowns with a composite resin. J. Prosthet. Dent. 45:455, 1981.
Reiss, R. Intraoral technic to repair veneer crowns and pontics. Dent. Surv. 49:41, 1973.
Richardson, J.T., et al. Repair technique for a fractured crowned tooth. J. Prosthet. Dent. 37:547–549, 1977.
Rochette, A.L. A ceramic bonded by etched enamel and resin for fractured incisors. J. Prosthet. Dent. 33:287–293, 1975.
Rouse, L.E. A technique for the repair of a fractured crowned tooth. J. New Jersey Dent. Assoc. 49:20–22, 1977.
Ruskin, A.R. In-the-mouth repair technic. Dent. Surv. 46:37, 1970.
Scimone, F.S. Chairside repair of porcelain fractures in bridgework. Dent. Surv. 52:42–49, 1976.
Silverman, G. Salvage and repair of fixed partial dentures I. Quint. Int. 10:49–53, 1979.
Watson, P.A. Treatment of porcelain fractures on metal ceramic splints. Ont. Dent. 53:7–8, 1976.
Ward, G.T., et al. Intraoral technic for repair of veneer facings. Ann. Dent. 36:35–40, 1977.
Welsh, S.L., et al. Repair technique for PFM restorations. J. Prosthet. Dent. 38:61–65, 1977.

Chapter 4

Restoration of Abutment Teeth Under Existing Partial Dentures

Many people wear removable partial dentures. The reasons for construction of a removable rather than a fixed restoration relates to the patient's periodontal condition, the numbers and/or locations of the missing teeth, the condition of abutment teeth, and financial considerations. In many of these cases, the denture will remain functional longer than one or more of the abutment teeth or the restorations on those teeth. This means that the dentist is often asked to restore an abutment tooth, and simultaneously maintain the serviceability of the removable partial denture.

Why does the denture remain functional for longer than the abutment teeth or the restorations? First is the question of treatment planning. In the interest of making conservative decisions, or saving the patient the expense of a crown, the dentist will often use a new or existing silver amalgam restoration on an abutment tooth which properly should be restored with some type of casting.

In the situation shown in Fig. 4-1, if a removable partial denture had to be made, most of the teeth that would serve as abutments would need to be restored with crowns. The only exception might be the maxillary right second molar, which could serve adequately even if a rest were placed on the tooth. None of the other teeth, however, should be left restored with intracoronal restorations if they are to be used as abutments.

Strength of abutment teeth

One criterion for restoration of abutment teeth for partial dentures is that the structural integrity of the remaining tooth can withstand both the magnitude and the vectors of force which will be applied when the removable partial denture is placed in function. When one considers the extra load that an MOD amalgam or inlay will be required to resist in the case of a distal extension partial denture with a mesial rest, the potential danger to that tooth is clear. The same tooth with normal occlusal function might not be at risk. However, by changing the loading and

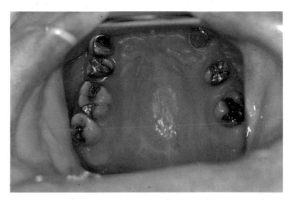

Fig. 4-1 Large silver amalgam restorations with too little integrity of remaining tooth structure for partial denture abutments.

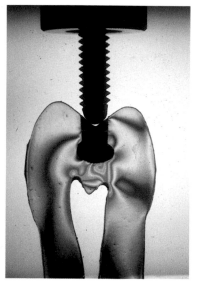

Fig. 4-2a Photoelastic specimen with inlay demonstrating adverse stress concentrations when loaded, as by an occlusal rest.

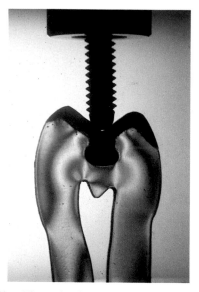

Fig. 4-2b Photoelastic specimen with onlay demonstrating better stress distribution when loaded similarly.

concentrating the force directly on an intracoronal restoration, especially one where both proximal surfaces have been weakened by the loss of sound tooth structure, there is a great risk of the tooth fracturing after a period. This is particularly true in the case of an MOD inlay where the concentration of force on a mesial or distal occlusal rest can increase risk of stress concentration in critical areas of the tooth, and predispose it to fracture (Figs. 4-2a and b).[1,2]

Another criterion is that the contours of the abutment tooth must fulfill the requirements for retention, correct path of insertion, and periodontal health. While sometimes it is preferable to make such an adjustment on the natural tooth structure, it is often necessary to construct a crown in order to attain the necessary parameters. These will be discussed later.

In summary, the abutment tooth and any restoration must not be at risk when put in service under the new partial denture, and the contour of the tooth must be correct to allow the partial denture to serve the patient adequately and to function according to accepted parameters.[3]

Defects in teeth or restorations

One reason for the difference in longevity between the removable partial denture, the abutment teeth, and associated restorations is that certain things happen to the abutment teeth which do not happen to dentures. Caries is one such occurrence. From a statistical standpoint, it is probably more likely that a tooth used as a partial denture abutment will be subject to recurrent caries more than a tooth in an ideal arch, all other things being equal.

The removable partial denture can make oral hygiene more difficult, if we can assume that it is unlikely that the denture will be removed and the teeth cleaned as often as recommended. In addition, the patient who has lost enough teeth to require this type of denture is probably a poor risk from the standpoint of oral hygiene. So, while we might not be addressing the same type of failure of the abutment tooth or its restoration, the tooth may still need a new crown because the margin of the old crown has become carious.

Because of defects in either the teeth or the restorations on them, corrective treatment is often needed. Unfortunately, the course of action too often followed results in making a new denture when the previous one could have been saved.

It would be ideal if the dentist had a workable method at his or her disposal for replacement of such a crown under the existing partial denture.

Treatment alternatives

There are essentially four alternatives for handling this problem:

1. Construct a new partial denture after restoring the tooth with a new crown.
2. Modify the existing partial denture to fit the new crown by making a new attachment for the partial denture.
3. Construct a new crown to fit the existing partial denture attachment.
4. Modify the partial denture by removing the involved attachment after construction of a new crown.

The advantage of making a new partial is that it is the best chance for an ideal result. The disadvantage is that it is the most expensive alternative.

There is another disadvantage to this alternative for many patients. It is not uncommon to treat a patient who has had many partial dentures made and is finally satisfied with the one they have now. In this situation, the dentist equipped with the best techniques will be able to allow the patient to keep their partial denture.

The primary advantage to modifying the existing partial denture by making a new retainer after the tooth has been restored is that the patient is able to retain the denture. There are two disadvantages, however. First, the patient must function without the partial while the laboratory procedure is being accomplished. Second, the laboratory steps are difficult, usually involving high-fusing soldering, or electrowelding, of nonprecious alloys.

There are many procedures advocated for constructing a new crown to fit the existing partial denture and the literature is replete with descriptions of such procedures. The greatest majority involve some type of a direct/indirect technique. In these methods, the pattern for the new crown is partially developed in plastic in the mouth, during which time the relationships between the tooth and the partial denture attachment are established. The rest of the pattern, namely the margins and other contours, are finished in the lab on a cast.[4-9] In other methods, the pattern is made entirely by the indirect procedure. In these, the removable partial denture must be kept in the lab as all the relationships are developed on the cast.[10-14] Several variations are presented in this chapter. Those that the authors consider the most dependable result in the best final fit of both crown and partial, and are relatively easy to accomplish. The success of these methods depends on the design of the partial and the skill of the dentist and technician. The primary advantages are cost, and the fact that it is not always necessary to make a new partial denture. The primary disadvantage to most of these methods is that the patient must function without the partial denture while the technician waxes the crown, and bakes the porcelain, if indicated. Some variations do not require the patient to function without the partial denture since they are basically accomplished directly.

Finally, the alternative of simply constructing a new crown and then removing the clasp from the partial denture is probably the easiest solution. However, the number of cases in which this will be possible or even desirable, is limited. Most partial dentures will need the retainers with which they were designed. There are, however, enough exceptions to make the method worth considering.

Principles of removable partial denture design

Before considering the various methods for restoring these abutment teeth, it might be wise to look at the principles that dictate the design of the retainer restorations in the first place. Obviously, our primary goal in these corrective procedures is to arrive at essentially the same form, fit, and function as the original tooth or restoration had. For example, frequently the patient will present with a design involving circumferential clasps rather than I bars. These cases may have no significant guiding planes, with most of the tooth preparation involving simply the occlusal rests. While most dentists would consider this less than ideal, many of these partial dentures are satisfactory, and it is in patients' best interests to maintain them. In such cases, the clinician must be familiar with the existing design, even though it is no longer commonly used.[15] The dentist sometimes can improve on the overall design of the partial denture in the process of making the correction, but in most cases it will be necessary to replace the crowns or the denture attachments with ones that match the original design.

It behooves us to consider the different partial denture designs that directly affect the process of making corrections, variations the dentist is likely to encounter, and how they affect treatment decisions.

Nature of the edentulous space

The first consideration is the number and location of missing teeth. The dentist will be faced with two options: either the case will be basically toothborne or it will involve a distal extension, or free-end saddle, as it is sometimes called. Toothborne cases are generally easier to handle when making corrections, just as they are easier to treat with partial dentures in the first place.

Remember that the partial denture will have a vertical surface that contacts with one or more areas on the old crown, be it natural tooth or restoration. The corresponding surfaces of the new restoration will need to fit those surfaces of the old partial denture. The dentist is allowed little creativity here, but not much is needed.

Distal extension cases are more complex to correct, especially in terms of the most distal, or terminal, abutment teeth. When these cases are properly designed and all of the procedures are done correctly, a certain amount of movement is allowed to take place between the framework and the abutment tooth. Remember again the basic premise here: *we are involved with making a restoration which is to fit and function with an existing partial denture*. Originally, the crown was made first; then the partial denture was made to function with it. In making a correction, the dentist will be called upon to reverse this procedure, making it extremely important that the operator fully understands the philosophy of the original design. He or she must also exert great care to construct the new restoration in a manner which will allow it to function with the old partial denture exactly the way the previous tooth contour did.

Retainers

Design features of removable partial dentures are crucial to the success of many facets of the restoration, such as proper occlusal plane, fulcrum line, and tissue-bearing surfaces. That part of the partial denture involving attachment to the abutment teeth is a primary concern. Again, it is essential that the dentist fully understand and appreciate the design parameters inherent in a particular restoration, even though the dentist may not ever have made a denture according to that design.

The most commonly used direct retainers are the suprabulge and infrabulge. A suprabulge retainer crosses the survey line as it approaches an undercut. Examples of the suprabulge are the circumferential or Akers, back-action, fishhook, and ring clasp (Fig. 4-3a). An infrabulge retainer approaches the crown from an apical direction. It does not cross the survey line. Examples of this retainer are the I-bar and T-bar (Fig. 4-3b).[16]

These various clasps were designed into the partial denture specifically for retention. When the crown is constructed under such an attach-

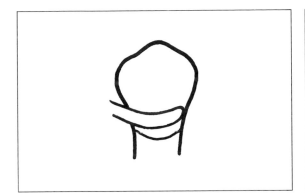

Fig. 4-3a Circumferential, or suprabulge, clasp.

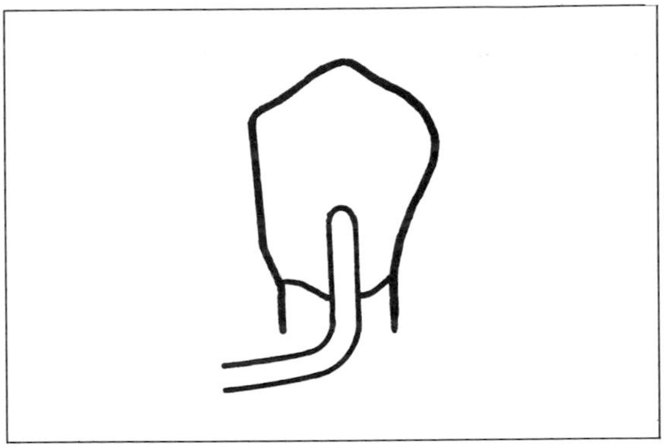

Fig. 4-3b I bar, or infrabulge, clasp.

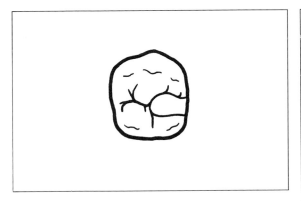

Fig. 4-4 Occlusal rest.

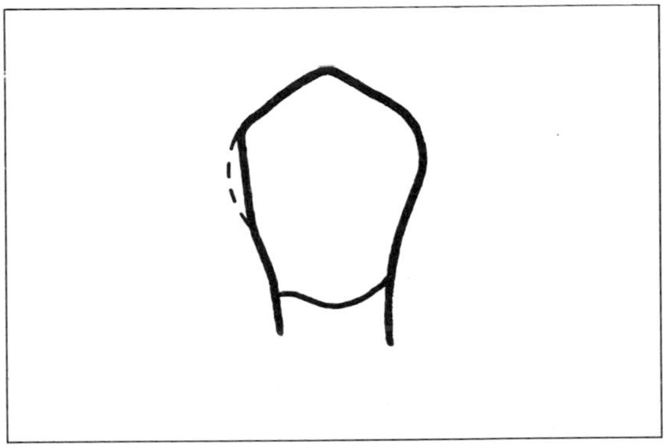

Fig. 4-5 Guiding plane.

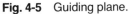

ment, all applicable parameters of the original form of the crown must be incorporated, or retention will be inadequate.

Rests and proximal plates must also be considered when constructing a crown under an existing removable partial denture. *Rests* provide resistance to movement in the direction of the supporting tissues (Fig. 4-4). *Proximal plates* of the partial denture framework fit against the guide planes of the abutment crown. Closely associated with the proximal plates are any other features of the design, such as lingual plates, that might be in contact with the new crown (Fig. 4-5). Since these two features are integral to the design of most partial dentures, they deserve a detailed examination.

Rests

The primary purpose of occlusal or incisal rests in partial denture design is to protect and maintain the integrity of the remaining oral structures. They should be positive, and at right angles to the directions of force applied to the abutment teeth by the partial frameworks. The rests must resist most of the forces applied to the denture in function, particularly those applied during mastication and during swallowing. In both situations, the forces are directed apically. If the denture had been originally designed such that the rest was on a large, weak, amalgam restoration, such a filling may have failed due to its inability to withstand such forces. The

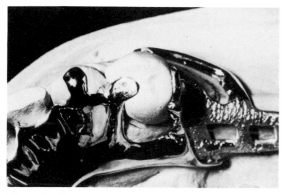

Fig. 4-6 Typical RPI attachment showing occlusal rest, proximal plate, and I bar.

design of the original rest must be correct—in terms of angle and size—or a new crown will simply repeat the same inadequate occlusal rest function.

Proximal plates

Proximal plates are used primarily in designs that also incorporate infrabulge retainers. This is known as the RPI design (Fig. 4-6). They present difficult problems to the dentist constructing a new crown under an existing partial denture. The plates approximate the axial surface of the abutment tooth next to the pontic area. Yet when the partial denture framework was initially constructed, the plate did not closely fit the surface of the crown over a great area. This is particularly true in the case of a distal extension design; in a toothborne partial denture the contact may be closer.

In distal extension cases, care should be taken to allow freedom of movement between plate and crown when the denture base is placed in function. Developing this relationship when the new crown is made to fit the partial denture is not an easy task. Proximal plates are considered so important by most teachers and practitioners today that their functions should be examined here.[17] They are as follows:

1. Maintaining arch integrity by anterior-posterior bracing action

2. Resisting dislodgement of the appliance by limiting movement away from the tissue
3. Acting as retainers by frictional contact with the paralleled guide planes
4. Protecting against food impaction by close fit with the guide planes
5. Maintaining soft tissue health at the tooth-tissue junction by functional contact, which prevents tissue hypertrophy or recession
6. Controlling tooth movement
7. Acting as a minor connector
8. Along with other minor connectors, reciprocating the retentive arm, thus generally eliminating the need for a reciprocating arm as with circumferential clasps

These proximal plates, in a removable partial denture which incorporates them, can present a problem for the dentist, and their importance cannot be overemphasized. Any attempt to construct a new crown under such a denture without adequately duplicating these features will produce an inferior fitting and poorly functioning restoration.

Construction of new crown with removable partial denture fitted to cast

Fitting a new crown to a removable partial denture on a cast requires that the patient be without the bridge during fabrication of the crown. If this is not feasible, then one of two actions must be taken: either some type of a temporary partial must be constructed, or an alternate technique will need to be employed to develop the contours of the restoration directly in the patient's mouth. The partial denture becomes an integral part of the model system on which the wax pattern, casting, and, if indicated, the porcelain procedures, will ultimately be carried out. There are some preconditions which must be satisfied before using this method:

1. The removable partial denture must have

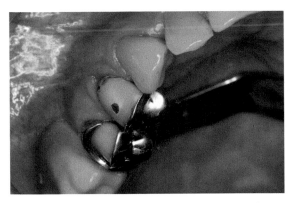

Fig. 4-7a Preoperative view of old plastic-faced crowns that no longer provide the needed undercut because of abrasion.

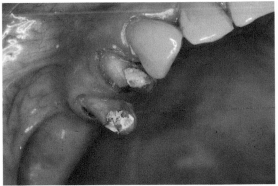

Fig. 4-7b Resulting preparations after removal of old crowns, ready for impressions.

an adequate number of abutment teeth, besides the one needing treatment, to stabilize the framework in the mouth. This is essential when we consider that the tooth to be restored under the existing framework was providing some stability, and was considered necessary in the original design. If this requirement is not satisfied, the technique should not be used.

2. If the framework does not fit perfectly, it must fit at least well enough to justify its acceptance during the initial construction of the case. The emphasis here is fit on the abutment teeth—the hard structures. It is irrelevant at this point whether the denture fits the residual ridges properly. A partial denture which needs a reline should be relined in any event. The fact that an abutment tooth needs to be restored under one of the attachments does not affect the efficacy of the reline procedure. In no instance should the tissue support, even if it is perfect, be relied upon to help relate the removable partial denture to the teeth.

3. The removable partial denture must be acceptable to the patient in all respects. For example, maintaining the existing partial is not indicated if the patient dislikes the shade of the teeth originally used.

4. Permanent features of the existing partial must be acceptable from a dental standpoint as well. These features include: vertical dimension of occlusion, centric position, tooth position, and placement and design of resistance and retention features.

Once these criteria have been met, fitting a new crown to an existing denture on a cast is in most cases the easiest and most reliable method for developing a wax pattern and baking porcelain under an existing attachment. Since the technician has the opportunity to place the partial onto the cast at will during the waxup and the porcelain application phases, the restoration can more easily meet the same high quality that the dentist would demand if the crown were being constructed prior to making the partial denture. As with all of the techniques described in this text, the goal is to arrive at a final result that is in all respects equal to or better than the original restoration.

Method

Step 1

Final preparation on the tooth may require removing a previous crown (Figs. 4-7a and b). For this procedure, refer to chapter 2. Endodontic procedures may also be needed in the case of a fractured tooth where it is no longer possible to achieve the same retention as for the previous crown. Developing the final preparation could

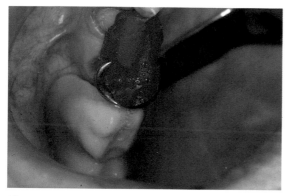

Fig. 4-8a Duralay index relating removable partial denture attachment to tooth in mouth.

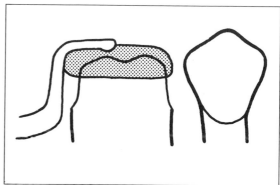

Fig. 4-8b Detail of index, demonstrating relationship of underside of rest to preparation.

also mean a buildup such as a dowel core, parapost buildup, or TMS pin buildup.

Step 2

Make impressions by one of the accepted methods. Note that while a dentist normally might use quadrant impressions, this technique requires that full-arch casts be generated. This is important because the dentist must be able to take advantage of the stability of the partial denture which is provided by contact between the attachments remote from the tooth being treated.

Ordinarily an impression might be accepted with minor flaws in areas that do not involve the preparation. In this case, however, any flaw in an area of contact between a hard tooth surface and the partial denture will usually dictate remaking the impression. It is essential that the denture fit *perfectly* on the full-arch cast. If it does not, then the contours of the new crown will be generated in an incorrect relationship to the rest of the dentition. When the crown is placed in the mouth, the denture will not be able simultaneously to seat on it and the rest of the abutment teeth.

Step 3

Using a plastic material such as acrylic resin, make an index of the relationship between the

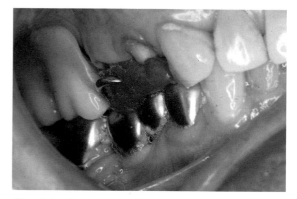

Fig. 4-9 Patient in CO with index and partial in place.

preparation and the partial denture attachment (Figs. 4-8a and b). Place the softened material over the occlusal surface of the preparation, covering no more than the occlusal one-third of the axial walls. Place the partial denture in the mouth and seat it completely onto the other abutment teeth. It will become obvious if insufficient stability is provided by the remaining abutment teeth to perform this technique. Finally, have the patient close into occlusion (Fig. 4-9). When the index has hardened, remove the denture and the index (Figs. 4-10a and b).

Step 4

Pour the impression to generate a full-arch

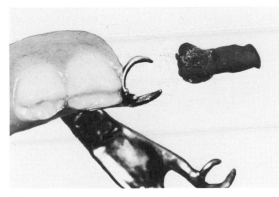

Fig. 4-10a Partial denture and index.

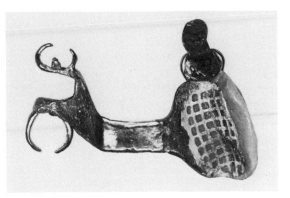

Fig. 4-10b Parts assembled ready for try-in on cast.

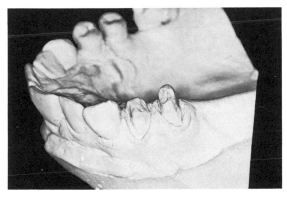

Fig. 4-11 Stone cast made from full-arch impression.

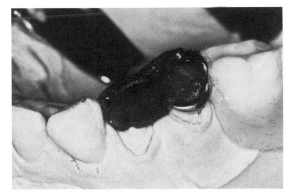

Fig. 4-12 Partial denture related to stone cast with plastic index.

working cast (Fig. 4-11). A solid cast can be made with separate finish line dies from a second quadrant impression, or a cast utilizing removable dies can be generated. The latter technique offers several practical advantages, and the likelihood of better results.

Step 5

Fit the partial denture to the cast with the aid of the plastic index. This is the most important step. The object is to adjust the cast in a manner as to allow the denture to be seated and removed at will, exactly as in the patient. This is accomplished by relieving any areas of the stone cast that interfere with seating of the denture onto the abutment teeth. An excellent means of doing this is with a red marking dye.* This means removing some of the stone which represents the soft tissues, such as gingival crests. It will seldom, if ever, be necessary to remove any stone representing hard structures, such as the abutment teeth. During this procedure, it is important to have the index in position to help orient the denture to the preparation (Fig. 4-12).

*Layout Fluid, Dayton Rogers Mfg. Co., Minneapolis, Minn.

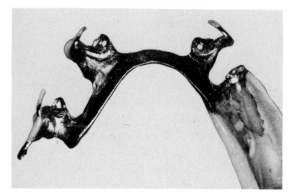

Fig. 4-13 Partial denture painted with red dye.

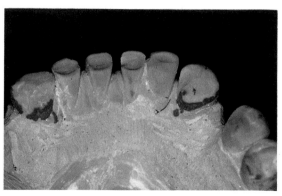

Fig. 4-14 Red dye transferred to cast indicating areas that are contacting.

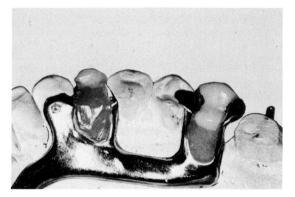

Fig. 4-15 Partial denture framework completely seated to tooth-bearing areas of the cast.

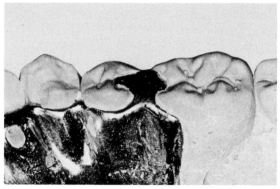

Fig. 4-16 Complex attachment showing double-occlusal rest, large lingual plate contact, and cingulum rest.

Step 6

Paint the inside of the partial denture framework with the dye (Fig. 4-13). This material will accurately transfer red marks onto the stone cast at points where the partial denture is prematurely contacting (Fig. 4-14). Progressively adjust the cast at the points of contact until the framework seats *perfectly* on all the abutment teeth (Fig. 4-15). Nearly all of the adjustment will be found in areas like the palate, facial flanges, and gingival crests. Observe the critical nature of this adjustment in Fig. 4-16, a case with a double occlusal rest, large lingual plates, and a cingulum rest on the canine. None of the tooth areas

needed to be adjusted, only the tissue areas. Figure 4-17 depicts the relationship on the cast between the I bar and the preparation.

In the solid cast method, separate impressions are made for two casts. One is an individual die for use in waxing margins, and the other is the solid full-arch cast.

Regarding the removable die method, a few comments on the design of the cast are necessary. The method the authors have found the most advantageous is the Pindex* system of cast construction. In this system, two or more pins are used in each removable section, fitting

*Whaledent International, New York, N.Y.

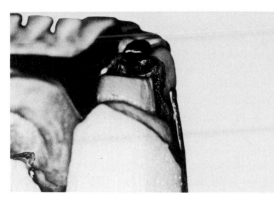

Fig. 4-17 Example of framework seated on working cast showing relationship of I bar to preparation.

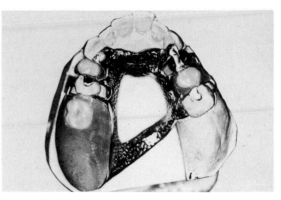

Fig. 4-18 Pindex system cast with partial denture seated.

into plastic sleeves rather than into holes in the stone itself (Fig. 4-18).

This removable die system results in accurate repositioning of the removable sections time after time. The most important thing to keep in mind here, while not applicable to most cases where this system is used, is to pin every edentulous area and each abutment tooth, not just the preparation. The use of this particular method will be dependent on its availability in the particular laboratory or dental office. Refer to chapter 9 for the specifics of the Pindex system.

The purpose of constructing the removable die cast by this method is to allow selective removal of the various sections of the cast as the partial is being fitted. Adjusting the cast to the partial framework is greatly simplified by this technique. It also allows a very simple way of pouring the stone so that the edentulous saddle areas of the partial denture are properly and positively supported.

Step 7

Pour any distal extension edentulous areas in new stone as follows:

1. Remove from the cast all existing distal extension edentulous areas just posterior to the last abutment tooth (Fig. 4-19).
2. Place new pins into the sleeves of the base.
3. Place the denture back onto the cast, after

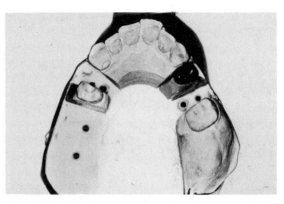

Fig. 4-19 Pindex system cast with some of the tooth and tissue areas removed, and with the wax pattern in place.

lubricating the inside of the saddle area with vaseline or tin foil substitute (Figs. 4-20a and b).
4. Secure the framework to the tooth areas of the cast where possible with sticky wax.
5. Box as needed to control flow of new stone.
6. Pour new stone into the denture saddle and around the new pins (Fig. 4-21). This will create a positive support for the distal extension area of the partial denture (Fig. 4-22). This is not likely to be the case if the original saddle area of the cast was used, as these cases are often in need of relining and lack a positive contact with the tissue. It must be understood that the new stone ridge is strictly a laboratory procedure, having noth-

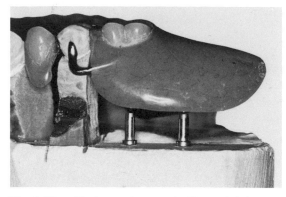

Fig. 4-20a Pindex system cast with partial denture in place and stone edentulous ridge area removed. New pins are in place and ready for pouring of substitute edentulous area for support.

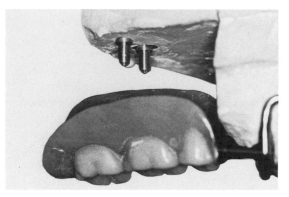

Fig. 4-20b Another example of the Pindex system, with different pin placement.

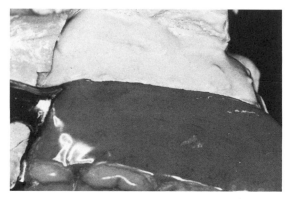

Fig. 4-21 Stone poured for substitute edentulous area.

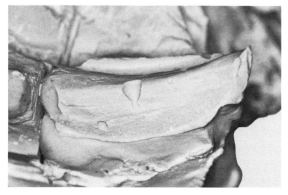

Fig. 4-22 Substitute edentulous area of cast that serves as support for the distal extension of the partial denture. Voids in stone are inconsequential as this is just used to support the saddle area on the articulator.

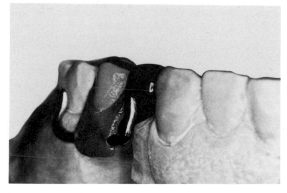

Fig. 4-23 Wax pattern on working cast with full contour in proper relationship to I bar.

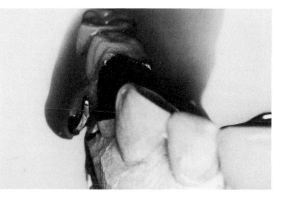

Fig. 4-24 Wax pattern on working cast after cutback for porcelain.

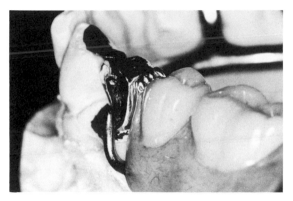

Fig. 4-25 Casting on transfer cast, ready for porcelain.

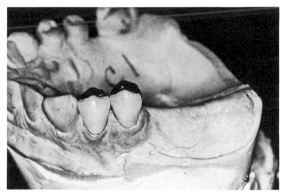

Fig. 4-26 Finished porcelain-fused-to-metal crowns on solid working cast.

ing to do with the fit of the partial to the ridge in the patient's mouth.

7. Again, keep the index in place throughout to help orient the partial to the preparation.

Step 8

An alternative method of creating this support for the saddle is simply to remove 2 to 3 mm of stone from the original edentulous area of the cast, moisten the cast, add a mix of new stone, then seat the partial denture. It should be pointed out that this method is more prone to inaccuracy than the former one. It is more applicable to the technique that uses a solid cast.

Step 9

Remove the index and partial denture and fabricate the wax pattern, taking special note of the following (Fig. 4-23):

1. Every time the partial denture is seated during the construction of the pattern, it must be seated all the way. If the wax is allowed to harden with the partial denture in a non-seated condition, then one of two things will occur on subsequent seatings: either the waxup will be "high," or it will crack.

2. The best way to ensure that the framework is seated each time is first to warm it with a flame; or the framework can be first placed into position, then seated by holding a warm

instrument against the attachment until it softens the wax.

Step 10

If the abutment restoration is to be a porcelain-fused-to-metal crown, then the cutback should now be made, with particular care taken to ensure adequate reduction of the wax for porcelain, and consideration given to whether the retentive clasp will necessarily limit freedom in this regard (Fig. 4-24). Now the casting can be made by normal technique.

Step 11

Try the casting on the working cast under the stereo microscope to verify the marginal fit. See chapter 9 for details on use of the stereomicroscope.

Step 12

Once the casting is seated, try the partial denture framework on the cast to verify that it seats perfectly, not only onto the stone abutment teeth, but also onto the new casting (Fig. 4-25).

Step 13

If the restoration is porcelain-fused-to-metal, the porcelain may now be baked (Fig. 4-26).

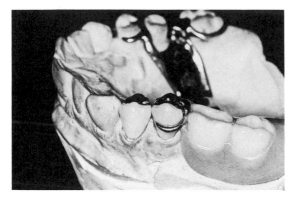

Fig. 4-27a Partial denture tried on the working cast, with new porcelain-fused-to-metal crowns ready for try-in in the mouth.

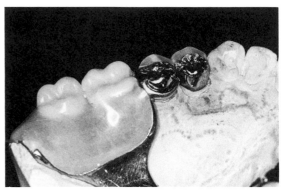

Fig. 4-27b Lingual view of partial denture on working cast with new crowns.

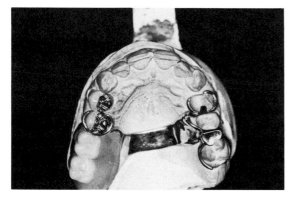

Fig. 4-27c Occlusal view of partial denture on working cast with new crowns. In this design, it is imperative that the framework perfectly fits the attachments on the contralateral side of the arch.

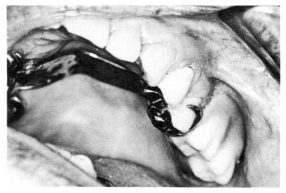

Fig. 4-28 Partial denture tried in the mouth with new crowns in place. Any discrepancy will usually require repeating the entire procedure, as it is nearly impossible to accommodate ill-positioning of the partial denture by adjustment.

Once this is done, the facial surface, now in porcelain, may be surveyed and adjusted to give the correct degree of undercut for the retentive clasp.

Step 14

Try the partial denture on the cast with the crown in place to verify the fit on all the other abutments as well as on the new restoration (Figs. 4-27a to c).

Step 15

Try the casting in the patient, using a silicone wash and inspecting for high spots under the stereomicroscope (Fig. 4-28). See chapter 9 for details on use of a silicone wash with the stereomicroscope.

Step 16

Once you are sure the crown is perfectly seated

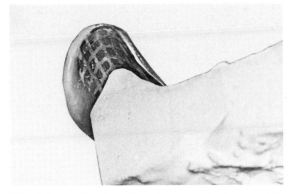

Fig. 4-29a Relationship of partial denture saddle area and cast during altered cast procedure, which was performed only on the distal portion of the saddle.

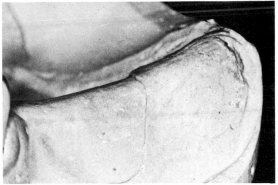

Fig. 4-29b Graphic demonstration of the need for a reline procedure, as seen by the change in level between the stone on the left, representing the ridge as it exists in the mouth, and the stone on the right, representing the actual tissue surface of the partial denture saddle. Note difference in height of stone.

to margin in the mouth—and only then—try in the partial denture. It must fit correctly onto all of the abutment teeth, including the new restoration. The crown can be temporarily cemented if it is necessary to verify the retention at this time. If everything fits well, this is usually not needed. Now cement the new crown, following normal techniques.

Step 17

The only remaining step will be eventual relining, if indicated. The altered cast referred to in step 7 would usually demonstrate whether or not a reline is needed (Figs. 4-29a and b).

Construction of new crown directly in patient using reinforced wax pattern

The primary difference between this method and the previous one is that in this case, the pattern is developed in the patient's mouth rather than in the laboratory. The advantage is that the patient may not need to function without

the partial denture. However, this is offset by some significant limitations. For example, since the wax pattern is actually developed in the mouth, it is not readily adaptable to situations where porcelain is involved in the areas of the crown contacted by the partial denture. Therefore, this method should be applied only to cases where the new crown is to be gold. Even though the failed crown may have been porcelain-fused-to-metal, the time since construction and placement may have altered the patient's perception of the need for such an esthetic restoration at present. Limitations of access and visibility in a given case will also play a role in whether to use this method. The same criteria listed earlier for acceptability of the removable partial denture apply to this technique, since the goals are the same—that is, that the previous partial denture be placed back in service after a new crown has been constructed.

Owing to these considerable limitations, and notwithstanding that the method presented here is common in the dental literature, it is presented here only as a secondary alternative. It should be attempted only when it is absolutely necessary for the patient to keep functioning with the old partial denture.

Method

Step 1

Complete tooth preparation. This may involve removal of the previous crown, a pin-retained buildup, or a post buildup. Whatever is indicated, arriving at a final preparation should be accomplished now.

Step 2

Make impressions with your preferred methods. As contrasted with the previous one, in this technique there is no relationship between the removable partial denture and the pattern during the laboratory phase. The cast produced will be used only for attaining proper occlusion and waxing the margins.

Step 3

The impression may be silver plated to make it more resistant to damage in subsequent steps. Or, it may simply be double-poured, providing that an impression material is used that has been shown to be accurate for second generation casts.

Step 4

Construct and place a temporary restoration for the tooth using the mold and core indirect temporary technique. For details of this technique, refer to chapter 9. The advantage of this technique is that it is the simplest and most dependable method for making a temporary crown that will allow the patient to continue to wear the partial denture during fabrication of the crown. There will be cases where, due to circumstances beyond the dentist's control, no method of generating a temporary crown will be satisfactory from the standpoint of retention, strength, and time. Patients in such cases will simply need to understand that they will be without the partial denture for a period, but that the laboratory phase will be completed as quickly as possible.

At this point, the dentist should lubricate the die with a tin foil substitute or a heavy die lubricant.

Step 5

Adapt a core of acrylic resin (Fig. 4-30). This is the central feature of the method, and carries the following requirements of the core:

1. It should be as thin as possible, not more than 1 mm at any point.
2. It should end at least 1 mm from the finish lines of the preparation. If possible, a greater distance should be left.
3. It must be stable on the die, but not exhibit any hint of binding, since the inner surface of the core will become the inner surface of the crown.
4. There must be clearance in the area of the occlusal surface, such that when the casts are in CO, there will be adequate room for wax.
5. Finally, and most importantly, this method is performed best if the entire outer surface of the pattern is to be in wax. No resin should be exposed. The authors feel that this will lead to the best result for the average clinician. It must be appreciated that any significant amount of finishing which must be done after casting to remove irregularities in the surface of the restoration will possibly alter an area which should be left untouched for proper fit of the partial denture framework.

Step 6

The patient needs to have a second appointment, during which the wax pattern is finalized. All of the outer contour that will involve the fit of the partial denture will be developed. The resin coping should be tried in and checked for stability on the preparation. The partial denture is then tried in over the coping to verify clearance in all areas between the two. Rest seats, guiding planes for proximal plates, and surfaces for retentive clasps should be generated in the wax portion of the pattern. Surfaces for retentive

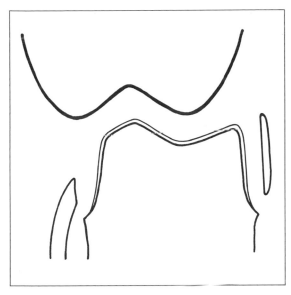

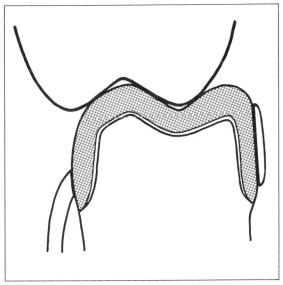

Fig. 4-30 Acrylic resin core on die in relation to lingual plate and I bar.

Fig. 4-31 Wax pattern developed to function with the various features of the partial denture attachment.

clasps are the most difficult part of this method because the dentist must develop the undercut itself in wax in the patient's mouth. As a reasonable compromise, if the surface for seating of the clasp is made correctly at this time, the contour occlusal to that area can later be generated on the mounted cast in the laboratory using a surveyor.

Replace the temporary crown in the patient. The following three steps are done in the laboratory:

Step 7

Wax the occlusion in a contrasting color on the mounted cast.

Step 8

Using a surveyor, carefully wax the indicated undercut by adding wax and carving it to proper form occlusal to the contact area of the retentive clasp arm. The degree of undercut will necessarily be determined by surveying the other undercuts and positioning the cast accordingly. When the partial denture was originally con-

structed, the dentist or the technician determined a line of draw for the denture. Many of the retentive areas now present in the case were then possibly developed in crowns. The pattern is thus completed (Fig. 4-31). At this point, we no longer have this freedom. We must generally accept the other undercuts and simply make the new crown fit into that scheme.

Step 9

In the laboratory, wax the margins of the pattern in a contrasting color wax (Fig. 4-32).

Step 10

The constrasting color wax in the two preceding steps allows the technician to avoid modifying any of the surfaces previously generated in the patient's mouth. It is easier to accomplish this goal by using a different color of wax for all laboratory work.

Step 11

Invest and cast the crown in the customary

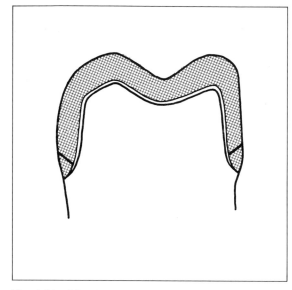

Fig. 4-32 Margins waxed in contrasting color wax.

manner. One advantage to having the complete outer contour in wax is now clear. Resin used in a pattern is known to burn out slower than the wax. If there were large areas of the pattern where the resin formed both the inside and the outside surfaces, that area of the mold could be blocked to timely evacuation of wax, often resulting in damage to the mold surface and resultant rough casting.

Step 12

Carefully polish the crown in preparation for try in. It is important not to overpolish, since all the surfaces involved in the fit of the partial denture must be left as undisturbed as possible.

Step 13

Try the crown in the patient's mouth and verify proper marginal fit, occlusion, and interproximal contours as with any crown. It is important to appreciate that although this restoration is constructed under an existing partial denture, the basic requirements of acceptability remain unaltered.

Step 14

Once it has been established that the crown will be acceptable, try in the partial denture. The following criteria must be met:

1. The partial denture must first seat all the way to its original position on all of the other abutment teeth without the patient feeling adverse pressure.
2. The partial denture must also fit the new crown in the areas of rest seats and guiding planes.
3. The partial denture must exhibit whatever degree of retention is required in each case. Bear in mind that the amount of retention required by the patient at this time may be less than before but that a certain amount of retention is mandatory.

Step 15

If any difficulty is encountered in seating the partial denture on the new crown, air brush the outer surface of the crown using aluminum oxide. Again try in the crown without cement and try in the partial denture. Then inspect the outer surface of the crown with a stereomicroscope for areas of hypercontact between the partial denture and the crown. Reduce these areas and repeat the process as necessary. Any technique for constructing a new crown under an existing partial denture has little or no room for error. In most cases, unless the partial denture seats perfectly the first time, the chances are that the crown will need to be remade.

Step 16

When all is in order, cement the crown in the usual manner. As with the previous method, the only remaining step is eventually to perform a reline if necessary.

References

1. Fisher, D.W., et al. Photoelastic analysis of inlay and onlay preparations. J. Prosthet. Dent. 33:47–53, 1975.
2. Fisher, D.W., and Caputo, A.A. An analysis of inlay and onlay design using three dimensional photoelasticity. Paper presented at the Annual Session of the American Association for Dental Research, New York, 1975.
3. Preston, J. Preventing ceramic failures when integrating fixed and removable prostheses. D. Clin. N. Am. 23:37–52, 1979.
4. Lee, R.E. Fabrication of a crown or inlay under an existing clasp. J. Wis. Dent. Soc. 46:221–223, 1970.
5. Samani, S.I., and Mullick, S.C. A new crown for an existing removable partial prosthesis. Quint. Int. 10:35–40, 1979.
6. Schneider, R.L. Adapting ceramometal restorations to existing removable partial dentures. J. Prosthet. Dent. 49:279–281, 1983.
7. Thurgood, B.W., et al. Complete crowns constructed for an existing partial denture. J. Prosthet. Dent. 29:507–512, 1973.
8. Welsh, S.J. Complete crown construction for a clasp bearing abutment. J. Prosthet. Dent. 34:320–323, 1975.
9. Gavelis, J.R. Fabricating crowns to fit clasp-bearing abutment teeth. J. Prosthet. Dent. 46:673–675, 1981.
10. Steinert, G. Full coverage for broken down partial denture abutments. Dent. Surv. 40:46–47, 1964.
11. Battistuzzi, P. The restoration of the abutment teeth under an existing removable partial denture II. Quint. Int. 5:17–28, 1974.
12. Fisher, F.J. The construction of cast crowns in relation to metal partial dentures. Br. Dent. J. 143:313, 1977.
13. Barrett, D.A., and Pilling, L.O. The restoration of carious clasp-bearing teeth. J. Prosthet. Dent. 15:309–311, 1965.
14. McLaughlin, G.T. Simultaneous crowning of abutments under existing prostheses. Dent. Surv. 47:24–25, 1971.
15. McCracken, W.L. Partial Denture Construction, 4th ed. St. Louis: The C.V. Mosby Co., 1977.
16. Berg, T.B. I-Bar: Myth and countermyth. D. Clin. N. Am. 23:65–75, 1979.
17. Kratochvil, F.J., and Vig, R.G. Principles of removable partial dentures (Unpublished syllabus).

Additional reading

Bartling, D. Preparation of a crown in the presence of an existing metal denture. Quint. Int. 3:27–28, 1972.

Battistuzzi, P. The restoration of the abutment teeth under an existing removable partial denture. I. Quint. Int. 5:17–28, 1974.

Brownfield, R.H. Full coverage for broken partial denture abutments. Dent. Surv. 39:50, 1963.

Chaney, S.A., and Thomas, D. Restoration of abutment teeth for an existing removable partial denture. Can. Dent. Assoc. J. 47:115–117, 1981.

Culpepper, W.D., and Moulton, P.A. Restoration of a crown to an existing removable partial denture clasp. D. Clin. N. Am. 23:30–35, 1979.

Ewing, J.E. The construction of accurate full crown restorations for an existing clasp by using a direct metal pattern technique. J. Prosthet. Dent. 15:889–899, 1965.

Garfield, R.E. Replacing an abutment crown for an existing removable partial denture. J. Prosthet. Dent. 45:37–43, 1981.

Goldberg, A.T., and Jones, R.D. Constructing cast crowns to fit existing removable partial denture clasps. J. Prosthet. Dent. 36:382–386, 1976.

Heintz, W.D. Treatment planning and design: Prevention of errors of omission and commission. D. Clin. N. Am. 23:3–12, 1979.

Hill, G.M. Construction of a crown to fit a removable partial denture clasp. J. Prosthet. Dent. 38:226–228, 1977.

Jackman, M.P., and Taylor, M.L. Crown construction to the lingual margin of a partial denture. Aust. J. Dent. 23:237–239, 1978.

Jordan, R.D. Multiple crowns fabricated for an existing removable partial denture. J. Prosthet. Dent. 48:102–105, 1982.

Kahl, R.E. A cast restoration to fit an existing partial denture. Dent. Dig. 69:250–253, 1963.

Killebrew, R.H. Crown construction for broken down partial denture abutments. J. Prosthet. Dent. 11:93–94, 1961.

Kratochvil, F.J. Five year survey of treatment with removable partial dentures. Part I. J. Prosthet. Dent. 48:237–244, 1982.

Loft, G.H., et al. An indirect method of crown fabrication for existing partial denture clasps. J. Prosthet. Dent. 38:589–591, 1977.

Lubovich, R.P., and Peterson, T. The fabrication of a ceramic-metal crown to fit an existing removable partial denture clasp. J. Prosthet. Dent. 37:610–614, 1977.

Moss, A.T. Case report: Saving crowns for a precision partial denture. Dent. Surv. 48:36, 1972.

Osborn, W.R. Full crown construction procedure for broken-down abutment teeth without altering partial denture. Dent. Surv. 40:58–59, 1964.

Reuter, J.E. Contingency planning in crown and bridgework design. Dent. Update 5:169–179, 1978.

Stamps, J.T., and Tanquist, R.A. Restoration of removable partial denture rest seats using dental amalgam. J. Prosthet. Dent. 41:224–227, 1979.

Teppo, K.W. A technique for restoring abutments for removable partial dentures. J. Prosthet. Dent. 40:398–401, 1978.

Warnick, M.E. Cast crown restoration of a badly involved abutment to fit an existing removable partial denture. D. Clin. N. Am. 14:631–644, 1970.

Wilsten, D. Direct pattern technique for crown fabrication under existing removable partial. J. Kan. St. Dent. Assoc. 64:14–15, 1980.

Chapter 5

Endodontic Procedures on Teeth With Existing Restorations

The increasingly high success rate of endodontic treatment has made it almost as routine as the silver amalgam restoration. Studies have reported success rates as high as 92% to 95%.[1,2] Many teeth have been saved that at one time would have been extracted, leading to masticatory systems that are in a considerably better state of health and function.

Owing to the high success rate of conventional endodontics, it should not be seen only as a last resort. Instead, with fixed prosthodontics, endodontic therapy may be beneficial prior to completing the final restorative treatment. In fact, high quality restorative dentistry may have been impossible in certain cases without endodontics, especially those cases with significant tooth structure loss due to caries or trauma.

It is sometimes advisable to perform endodontics prior to restoring the teeth even though the treatment may not be mandatory. For example, if a tooth is to be used as an abutment for a multiple-unit fixed bridge it may have had a previous large amalgam filling or crown. Although only minor or inconsequential symptoms may have been manifested, endodontics prior to seating the fixed restoration may be advisable in light of the danger to the retention of the restoration if the endodontics is attempted after the bridge is cemented. The same level or frequency of symptoms might not be treated but simply observed when a tooth does not need such a restoration.

Another situation in which endodontics prior to restoration should be considered arises when a single unit is prepared for a crown and impressions have been made. While the temporary is in place, mild tooth sensitivity can occur. The dentist determines that the temporary is not the cause, and a dilemma presents itself. This tooth has now undergone a series of insults to the pulp, and it may be prudent for the dentist to have endodontics performed now, rather than later, which would jeopardize the final restoration and put the patient through an extended period of uncertainty. In this instance, improved visibility allows more conservative access to the pulp chamber and canal than when the restoration is already in place.

While the indiscriminate use of endodontic therapy is unwise, there are cases where performing this treatment prior to placing an extensive or expensive restoration is not only justified, it is the treatment of choice. The dental pulp in a fully erupted and developed tooth has little practical use. Its part in formation of the root by virtue of the odontoblastic layer has been successfully completed years before, and its value as a defense mechanism owing to the presence of free nerve endings is questionable, particularly when patients seek regular dental care. However, a patient sometimes declines to have an endodontic procedure, even though the dentist recommends it. Some reasons for this are:

1. The symptoms or clinical and radiographic signs are not conclusive enough for either the patient or the dentist to take a firm stand on the necessity of the procedure.

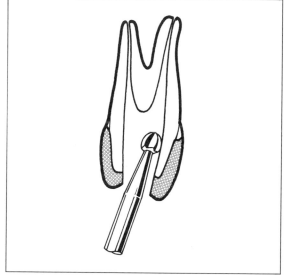

Fig. 5-1 The access must be of adequate size so as to allow a direct approach to all parts of the pulp chamber.

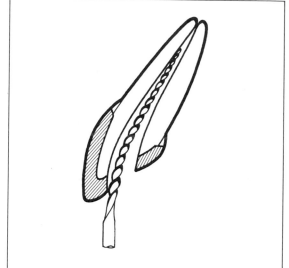

Fig. 5-2 If the access is made such that the file must bend to reach the apical area, the larger and stiffer files will tend to create a ledge in the wall of the canal.

2. The cost of the endodontic treatment, in addition to restoration costs, often makes it preferable for the patient to avoid the procedure if it is not absolutely necessary.
3. On occasion a patient will present for treatment with the preconceived notion that endodontic therapy is somehow not in their best interests due to their own or another's previous unfortunate experience.

None of the aforementioned reasons would be a justification for avoiding an endodontic procedure when the dentist is certain it is needed. They would apply only where the dentist is uncertain that the procedure is mandatory.

Relationship of preparation design to the problem

Consider the principles of attainment of endodontic access:

1. The access must be large enough to assure removal of all tissue from the pulp chamber, root canal, and coronal portion of the tooth (Fig. 5-1).
2. The access must be positioned in such a manner as to allow for a relatively direct entry with files into the pulp canal, that is, the radicular portion of the tooth. It is more important for the file not to be forced to bend in the coronal area of the tooth than in the apical area, because the file is much stiffer in the coronal area than near the tip (Fig. 5-2). If there is a relatively gentle curvature near the apex, the more flexible file tip will usually follow it. But if the file must bend in the thicker and more resistant area near the handle, there is going to be a greater effect on the actual control of the cutting action.[3]

Important design requirements for crown preparations

One or both of the above requirements may deviate from ideal preparation design. A look at a few of the requirements for preparations shows where conflicts might arise:

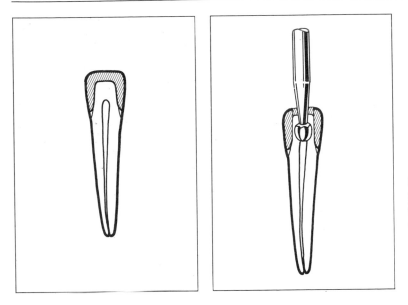

Fig. 5-3a (*far left*) A typical porcelain-fused-to-metal crown and the attendant preparation.

Fig. 5-3b (*left*) The problem caused by making an access in the restoration.

1. Parallelism of opposing walls

From a retention standpoint, it is essential that a preparation for a full crown have adequate parallelism between opposing facial and lingual walls, as well as the mesial and distal. These opposing walls must also have adequate length. If an endodontic access must be made in a tooth which has or will receive a crown, it is not at all inconceivable that one or more of these important walls might be compromised after the two procedures are accomplished (Figs. 5-3a and b). This problem is seen very graphically in the photographs showing a round bur and a typical preparation for a porcelain-fused-to-metal crown (Fig. 5-4).

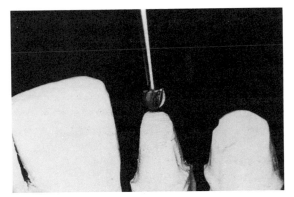

Fig. 5-4 A round bur of the size often recommended for making access in lateral incisors is seen to be large enough in relation to a typical crown preparation to likely compromise retention of the crown.

2. Strength of dentin

The remaining dentin comprising the preparation must be strong enough for the given situation, considering the occlusal forces to which the restoration will ultimately be subjected.

This requirement for strength of the remaining tooth structure will be considerably compromised where both a full crown preparation and

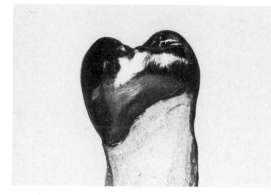

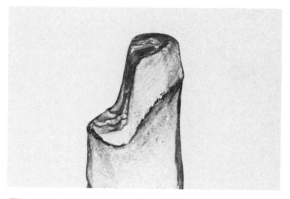

Fig. 5-5a A typical-appearing full gold crown on a premolar.

Fig. 5-5b The preparation which was actually under this relatively normally contoured crown.

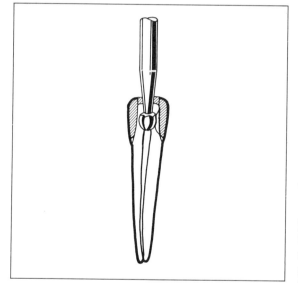

Fig. 5-6 The situation in which a small anterior tooth has lost a great amount of tooth structure because the porcelain-fused-to-metal preparation combined with the old mesial filling.

endodontic access opening have been performed on the same tooth. It will be further compromised if one or more of the retentive walls had been violated even prior to making the crown, such as where large mesial and distal plastic restorations existed (Figs. 5-5a and b). This is very common in small anterior teeth which have had deep mesial or distal restorations prior to placement of the crown (Fig. 5-6).

3. Parallelism of teeth

Bridge preparations can present additional problems. When looking at the retainer restorations in the mouth or on the diagnostic cast, the axial contours and occlusal anatomy may be such that the teeth appear in good alignment. This was usually the objective of the dentist and the technician when the restoration was originally made. However, often the teeth under these seemingly well-aligned retainers are not anywhere near parallel, sometimes having long axes which are 10° to 40° divergent.

The advisability of constructing fixed bridges with this kind of extreme divergence is outside of the scope of this text, especially the problem caused by adverse loading of the periodontal ligament on the mesial aspect of the roots. Here we are concerned with an otherwise successful restoration in which this condition already exists. Radiographs showing the alignment of the

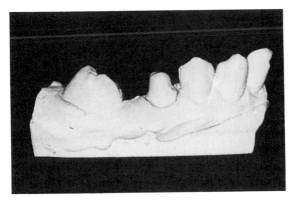

Fig. 5-7a Cast of a three-unit mandibular posterior bridge case with a typical tilted molar abutment. The premolar has been prepared in the prevailing line of draw for the bridge.

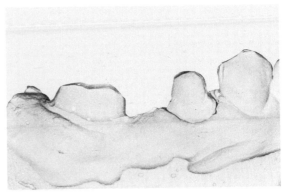

Fig. 5-7b The molar has now been prepared in this prevailing line of draw, grossly altering the relationship between preparation and the external contours of the crown that will eventually be placed on it.

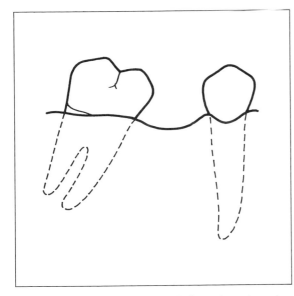

Fig. 5-8a Natural anatomy of a tipped molar abutment.

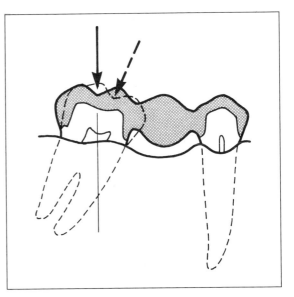

Fig. 5-8b Resulting anatomy of the final restoration. The broken arrow shows the correct access location, and the solid arrow shows what would appear to be the correct access location if only the new occlusal anatomy is considered.

roots are invaluable (Figs. 5-7a and b). Figure 5-8 shows the final contour of the bridge retainer in relation to the original contour of the tipped molar abutment. One can appreciate the potential difficulty of locating the canals using the anatomical landmarks presented by the restoration as a guide (Figs. 5-8a and b).

4. Original working cast

This is an area where the original working casts showing the preparations themselves are the best aid the dentist could hope for. If these are available, the dentist or the endodontist has information which could easily make the differ-

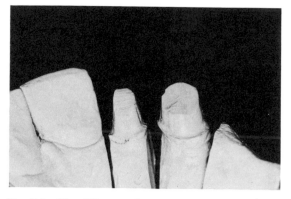

Fig. 5-9 The difference in preparation size between a typical maxillary lateral incisor and a maxillary canine. The amount of tooth structure available for making access without compromising the retention of a crown varies greatly.

ence between saving or losing the tooth or the restoration when endodontics is performed (Fig. 5-9).

Dimensions of access and burs

How large does the access need to be? Many sources can be consulted in coming to an agreement on the size of the bur to be used in making the access opening for an endodontic procedure. A review of the literature shows burs ranging from nos. 2, 4, or 6 round[4] to nos. 8 or 11 round[5] depending on the size of the tooth. It is significant to note that it is the smaller end of this spectrum that is recommended by more contemporary authors. The decrease in size is commensurate with a much greater appreciation on the part of both general dentists and endodontists over recent years of a need for conserving tooth structure when performing access openings.[6,7]

Looking at the relationship between preparation size and bur size, it is evident that in many situations it will be difficult if not impossible for even the most experienced endodontists, exercising the utmost in care, to avoid compromising, if not destroying, the integrity of the crown preparation. Table 5-1 indicates this relationship, taking into account the average size of typical clinically acceptable preparations. The figures for preparation size are for the dimension of the preparation at a point one-half the distance between the incisal or occlusal surface and the gingival finish line of the preparation. The smallest dimension is the limiting factor, in that if the bur approaches that size, there is danger of removing a retentive wall.

These measurements do not take into account the fact that in actual practice, there is likely to be more tooth structure removed during access preparation than just the diameter of the bur. This is because the operator does not have the natural anatomic landmarks of the normal unmodified occlusal surface as a guide, and the fact that there is always a certain amount of nonconcentric action of the bur.

The problem is more acute in the anterior teeth, or in small premolars than in molars, even though a larger bur is used in the latter (Figs. 5-10a and b). Therefore, the size and geometric form of the crown preparation is to be considered when endodontic therapy is needed. The following could apply in this area:

1. If a restoration is already in place when the need for endodontic treatment becomes evi-

Table 5-1 Relationships of typical endodontic preparations to recommended access burs.

Tooth	Recommended bur	Size of bur (mm)	Size of preparation (mm)
Mandibular anteriors and maxillary premolars	nos. 2–6	1–1.8	3.0–3.7
Maxillary anteriors and mandibular premolars	nos. 4–6	1.4–1.8	3.25–3.5
Molars	nos. 6–11	2.3–2.7	7.0

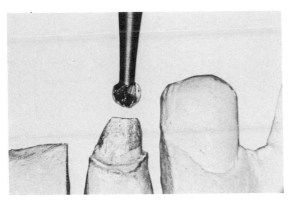

Fig. 5-10a A round bur positioned to make access showing the relationship of the bur to the size of a premolar preparation.

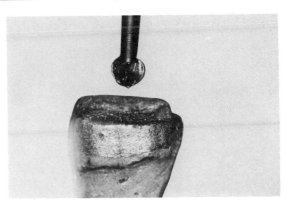

Fig. 5-10b Use of the same bur showing the greater amount of tooth structure available in a molar for making a safe access without destroying the retention of a crown.

dent, how likely is it that the retention, and possibly the tooth, might be lost if conventional endodontics were done through the existing crown?

2. If eventual endodontic treatment is considered a possibility, albeit a remote one, and the restoration is not yet cemented on the tooth, precautions should be taken to ensure the greatest probability of success.

Casting design when endodontics might be needed in the future

Currently, a high percentage of fixed prosthodontic restorations are full crowns with porcelain coverage. The extent varies from the facial surface only, as on many maxillary posterior teeth, to full coverage on mandibular posterior teeth where the occlusal surface is often covered with porcelain for maximum esthetics. This presents a serious problem when such a restoration needs to be penetrated from the occlusal surface in order to attain endodontic access. Such an opening in the occlusal surface of a porcelain-fused-to-metal restoration may give rise to the potential for fracture and/or loss of the bond between the porcelain and the metal coping because of the adverse distribution of stresses.

Where a restoration is yet to be cemented, it is possible to take precautions in the design to allow for future access to the pulp canal without loss of the restoration or the abutment tooth. Two avenues are available: either the original design of the porcelain coverage can be modified to make future access easier, or premade access can be incorporated into the design of the casting. For example, instead of full porcelain coverage on a mandibular premolar, a metal occlusal surface can be used, with only the facial surface and tip of the functional cusp in porcelain (Figs. 5-11 and 5-12). There will be only metal in the area where the endodontic access would be made, if it is ever necessary (Figs. 5-13a and b). The same principle can be followed with anterior teeth, with greater lingual coverage in metal (Figs. 5-14a to c).

When the potential for future endodontic treatment is considered more likely, and it is not done prior to cementation, a procedure can be followed that will result in a premade access. This technique involves placing a cast gold inlay in access. The following section describes this technique in detail.

Method: Cast gold inlay

Step 1

The crown or bridge retainer is designed with a

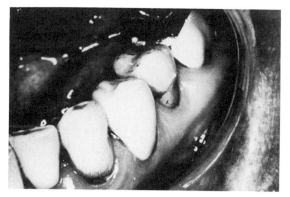

Fig. 5-11 Porcelain-fused-to-metal crown on a mandibular first premolar with porcelain occlusion.

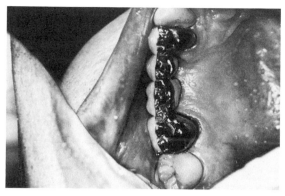

Fig. 5-12 Maxillary restoration showing gold occlusion, allowing access without compromising the integrity of the bond or the porcelain.

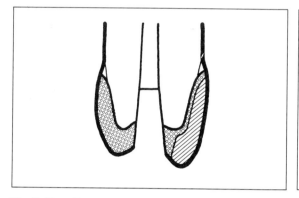

Fig. 5-13a Porcelain-fused-to-metal crown with full porcelain occlusion.

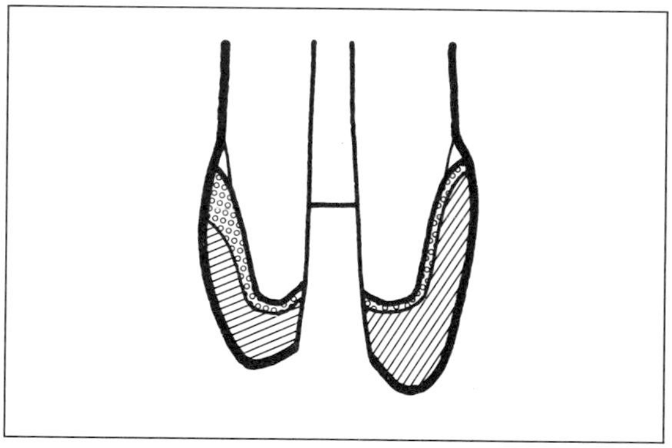

Fig. 5-13b Porcelain-fused-to-metal crown with gold occlusion.

metal occlusal surface, ensuring that the coverage of porcelain on the facial cusp tip is extensive enough to satisfy only the requirements for stress distribution related to bond strength. If the restoration contemplated is to be a gold crown with no porcelain coverage, then this requirement will be automatically satisfied.

Step 2

Using the radiographs, diagnostic cast, and working cast of the finished preparation, determine the location of the endodontic access on the occlusal surface of the preparation as though it were to be done now through the preparation (Fig. 5-15).

Step 3

Transfer this location visually to the inside of the new cast restoration and mark with a pencil (Fig. 5-16). Working from the inside of the casting, make an opening just the size of the contemplated access (Figs. 5-17a and b). Place the crown with the premade access opening on the tooth (Fig. 5-18).

Step 4

After adequate anesthesia is attained, finish the resulting Class I occlusal preparation by extending it into the dentin of the tooth to attain adequate retention for the forthcoming restora-

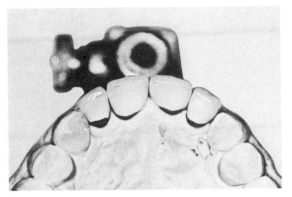

Fig. 5-14a Porcelain-fused-to-metal crowns on maxillary centrals and laterals designed with porcelain lingual surfaces.

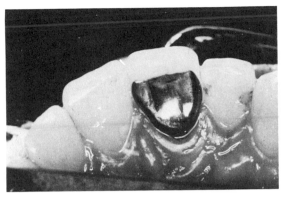

Fig. 5-14b A porcelain-fused-to-metal crown with gold lingual surface.

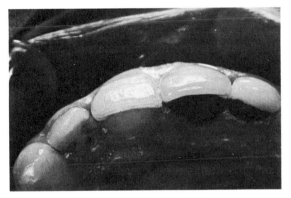

Fig. 5-14c A view more in line with the long axis of the tooth indicates the increased ease that such a design provides when trying to make access into the canal.

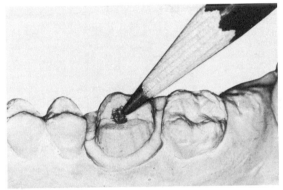

Fig. 5-15 Anticipated location of future endodontic access, should one become necessary, being plotted on the cast.

tion. Develop the outline of a typical small Class I preparation during this step.

Ensure that the preparation outline has some irregularly, rather than perfect roundness since this will aid in orienting the inlay on seating. Flare the preparation following normal preparation design principles for attaining retention and finishing bevels. If the occlusal reduction of the crown preparation is great enough to allow for walls at least 2 mm long, then the entire preparation will be done in the crown with the floor being the occlusal surface of the crown preparation. More often than not, however, it will be necessary to extend the preparation into the dentin of the tooth 1 or 2 mm (Fig. 5-19). The

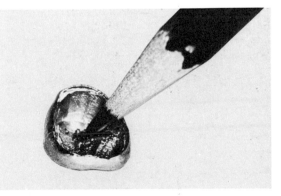

Fig. 5-16 Location of access transferred to the inside of the crown.

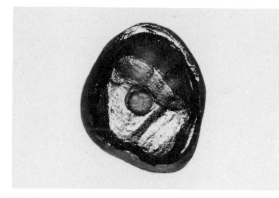

Fig. 5-17a View from inside the crown showing the access opening.

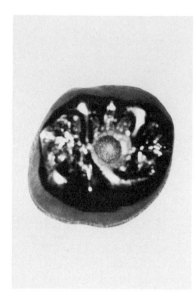

Fig. 5-17b View of the access opening from the occlusal surface.

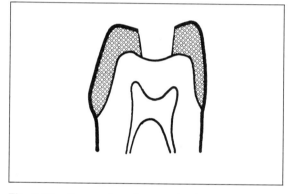

Fig. 5-18 Crown placed on tooth with access opening as shown in Figs. 5-17a and b.

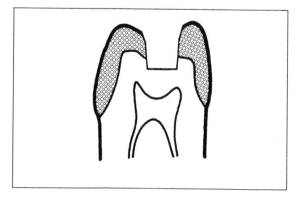

Fig. 5-19 The final Class I inlay preparation is developed in the crown and the dentin together, including the occlusal bevel.

crown now has the upper half of a modified Class I inlay preparation (Fig. 5-20). It is unnecessary to extend the outline into all of the occlusal grooves since this surface is cast gold, not natural enamel.

Step 5

Remove the crown from the preparation, and examine the depression in the dentin that resulted from the extension of the preparation into the tooth. If possible, have an endodontist verify the position of the access in relation to the pulp canal. Simply make a small quadrant alginate impression of the tooth, pour it in fast-setting plaster, and show this to the endodontist, cementing the crown at a later appointment.

Step 6

The crown can be cemented after determining that the preparation into the tooth is correctly placed.

Step 7

The inlay can be made either by a direct wax pattern, or by making an impression and doing an indirect pattern. This can be simply a quadrant impression done with a double-bite technique. The method for constructing the inlay is discussed on page 105. The technique for using the Check Bite tray is described in chapter 9. Opposing casts are quickly generated and are more than adequate for the restoration. Clear the cement from the access opening in the crown, and temporize the area while the inlay is being made. Cement the inlay at a subsequent appointment.

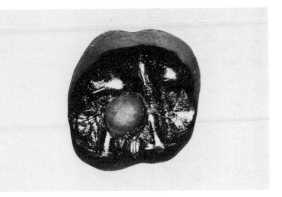

Fig. 5-20 Crown with final modified inlay preparation.

Step 8

If it is necessary to perform endodontic treatment on the tooth at a later time, it will be relatively easy to gain proper access to the canal because the inlay gold is softer than that of the crown. The endodontist should be able to gain access without destroying the underlying crown preparation, as often ensues when the exact location of the pulp chamber in relation to the occlusal anatomy of the casting is unknown.

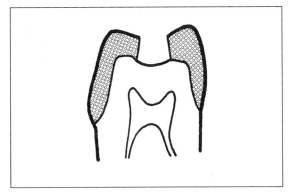

Fig. 5-21 Crown in place on tooth with the portion of the access completed that is just in the crown.

Method: Direct gold foil

Step 1

Design the restoration with a metal occlusal surface, and ensure that the coverage of porcelain on the facial cusp tip is only extensive enough to satisfy the requirements for stress distribution related to bond strength. If the restoration contemplated is to be a gold crown without porcelain coverage, then this requirement will be automatically satisfied.

Step 2

Use the radiographs, diagnostic cast, and working cast of the finished preparation to determine the location of the endodontic access on the occlusal surface of the preparation as though it were to be done now through the preparation (Fig. 5-15). Transfer this location visually to the inside of the new cast restoration and mark it with a pencil (Fig. 5-16).

Step 3

Working from the inside of the casting, make an opening only the size of the contemplated access (Figs. 5-17a and b). Place the crown with the premade access opening on the tooth (Fig. 5-18).

Step 4

Undercut the preparation for retention. This presents one minor problem, in that normally a gold foil restoration to some extent depends on the elasticity of the dentin for starting retention, but here most of the axial wall area is the gold casting. Whenever possible in this instance, continue the extension into the tooth to the upper 1 to 2 mm of the coronal tooth structure. This should provide enough dentin wall surface area for retention (Fig. 5-21).

Step 5

Remove the crown from the preparation, and examine the small depression in the dentin, which resulted from the extension of the preparation into the tooth, for accuracy of location. Have your endodontist examine it if possible, since he or she is more experienced in judging correctness of the position in relation to the pulp canal. This will not usually be done, but it is a good idea when practical. However, it is often adequate to make a small quadrant alginate impression of the tooth, pour it in fast-setting plaster, show this to the endodontist, and cement the crown at a later appointment.

Step 6

Cement the crown after determining that the extension into the dentin is properly located. When gold foil is being used for a Class I restoration, it is usually safer to temporize the preparation at this point and condense the foil at a subsequent appointment. Otherwise condensation may disturb the new cement seal of the crown.

Step 7

If it is necessary to perform endodontic treatment on the tooth, it will be relatively easy to gain proper access to the canal because the gold foil is softer than the crown. Because of these precautions, the endodontist should be able to gain the access without destroying the preparation, which may occur if the exact location of the pulp chamber in relation to the occlusal anatomy of the casting is unknown.

Restoring access openings in existing restorations

It is common for a general dentist to be called upon to restore an access opening after an endodontist has completed treatment of the canal. The procedure is very similar to that of the premade access opening in a cast restoration. However, there are enough differences to warrant some discussion here.

The likely choices of materials are: silver amalgam, gold foil, composite resin, and cast gold inlay.

Dentist and patient alike often prefer to fill the access with silver amalgam. This is an inexpensive method, and requires just one appointment. In most cases, this method is acceptable, because if the access was done by an experienced endodontist, it will usually be small enough to involve little or no occlusal contact.

However, in many cases, the access is not small enough to meet this idealistic criterion. In these cases the authors recommend the defects be restored using a cast gold inlay. Since the preparation is flared, direct occlusal forces will not be able to dislodge it in an apical direction. Often with the silver amalgam or gold foil restorations in these cases because the preparation is undercut rather than flared, occlusal forces are able to drive the "filling" into the preparation. This results from the fact that in an endodontically treated tooth, there is often no solid dentin floor to the preparation as would be in a vital tooth. Instead, the floor of the preparation is made up of either gutta-percha, or some type of cement. Because of this, the endodontist should fill the coronal portion above the orifice of the canals with a crown-buildup composite material, rather than gutta-percha or cement. If there are some contact areas between the dentin and the composite, this results in a more structurally sound base no matter what type of restoration is used to seal the access in the existing restoration.

Method: Direct filling using silver amalgam, gold foil, or composite

Step 1

After the patient returns from the endodontist, the dentist should examine the access cavity after cleaning out the portion that involves the crown (Fig. 5-22). If the endodontist has filled the access with a composite plastic, which would have been ideal, then all that is needed is for the dentist to perform a direct filling preparation into the tooth structure, using the composite plastic as the floor of the preparation as described below. If the endodontist has filled the area of the access above the orifice of the canal with gutta-percha or cement, then it is advisable to replace this material with a crown-buildup type of composite plastic.

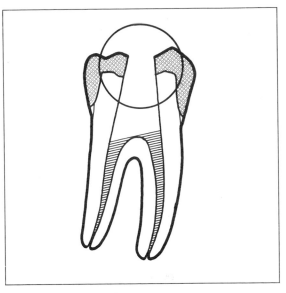

Fig. 5-22 Tooth with access through crown and into chamber, ready for composite base.

Step 2

Prepare a typical Class I cavity preparation with the relationships of the various materials as shown in Fig. 5-23. Note that the walls of the preparation will be undercut for retention and will be made of the gold and/or porcelain material in the occlusal portion and the dentin of the existing tooth more apically to that. The floor will be the composite plastic material (Fig. 5-23).

Step 3

Place the direct filling material after placing the rubber dam, and finish according to standard procedures.

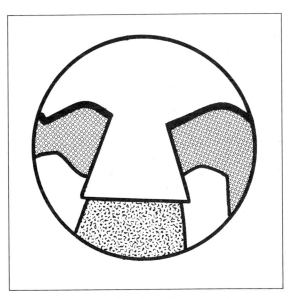

Fig. 5-23 Preparation through access incorporating: *(1)* undercut walls, *(2)* extension slightly into tooth structure, and *(3)* floor made of composite.

Method: Cast gold inlay

Step 1

After the patient returns from the endodontist, the dentist should examine the access cavity after cleaning out the portion that involves the crown (Fig. 5-22). It should be adequately filled up to the level of the proposed pulpal floor of the

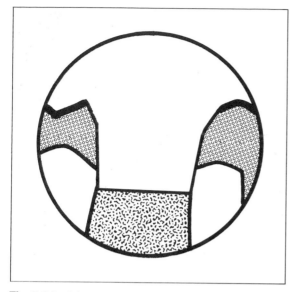

Fig. 5-24 Inlay preparation in access extending far enough into the underlying base to provide enough wall for retention.

preparation. In contrast to the direct filling method, it is not really important whether the area above the orifice is filled with gutta percha or a plastic material because this method is based on a flared preparation. Any occlusal force on the Class I restoration will be resisted by the gold crown rather than the underlying filling material.

Step 2

Complete the Class I inlay preparation in the crown and the underlying dentin as in Fig. 5-24. The parameters of this preparation are similar to the direct filling method, with the following significant exceptions:

1. The walls must be flared, not undercut.
2. The length of the walls is more critical than in the direct method. Retention is dependent on the length of the walls and this is even more important than for most Class I inlays because the endodontic access is more conservative—smaller in diameter—than that of the typical preparation.

3. While the endodontic access will usually be essentially round, it is best to develop some irregularity in the outline form of the inlay preparation. A perfectly round preparation will make it difficult to align the inlay at the time of seating and can reduce resistance to dislodgement. Making the preparation oval or triangular will solve these problems.

Step 3

Make an impression following normal practice. In a great many cases, this can be simply a quadrant impression done with a double-bite technique. In this manner, opposing casts are generated quickly that are more than adequate to provide all the parameters needed for such a restoration. Of course, as is the case with the technique for a premade endodontic access, a direct wax pattern could be developed if the dentist is so inclined. The Class I preparation will need to be temporized using a standard cement while the laboratory steps are being done. The inlay will be tried in and cemented following normal procedure at a subsequent appointment (Figs. 5-25a and b).

Method: Composite in anterior teeth with three-quarter crowns

Three-quarter crowns present a special problem. In contrast to a full gold or porcelain-fused-to-metal crown, there is the potential for esthetic degradation after the endodontic treatment. In a partial veneer crown, the facial surface of a maxillary central, for example, is uncovered. A metallic filling, particularly silver amalgam, can discolor the facial enamel. Therefore, it is recommended that these access openings be filled with an composite technique.

Step 1

Place a rubber dam. Clean out the entire chamber down to the cervical line and remove all root canal sealer.

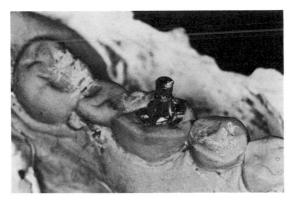

Fig. 5-25a Inlay on cast in access preparation.

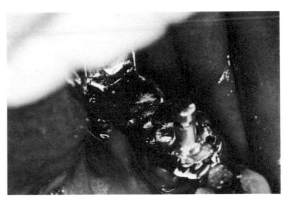

Fig. 5-25b Inlay tried in the crown in the mouth.

Step 2

Fill the chamber with an appropriate shade of composite. Experimentation may be needed to select the correct shade, since these materials were meant to be viewed when picking up the color of the adjacent tooth structure. It is the tooth structure which is visible; the composite material is the backing. When the correct shade has been selected, place the filling by normal means, and finish the composite on the lingual side as with any direct filling (Fig. 5-26).

Endodontic surgery and existing restorations

One of the most perplexing problems in dentistry is the development of a periapical lesion on an abutment tooth for a complicated or extensive prosthodontic restoration. Often the tooth involved is the abutment for a porcelain-fused-to-metal fixed bridge, or a critical abutment for a removable partial denture. Either situation presents the following dilemma:

1. The need to separate the patient from his or her disease is absolute.
2. The restoration may be perfectly satisfactory, may have cost the patient a great deal of time and money originally, and is sure to cost much more now.

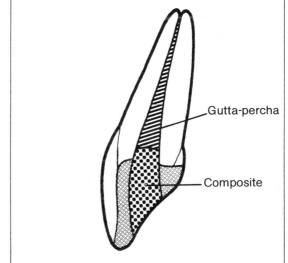

Fig. 5-26 Anterior tooth with three-quarter crown leaving facial enamel exposed. This situation is best restored by filling the chamber and the access with composite for the best and longest-lasting esthetic result.

Gutta-percha

Composite

3. For any number of reasons, the patient may want to save the restoration even if that means surgery is required.
4. The dentist and/or the endodontist may have reservations about the advisability and prognosis for attaining the endodontic access without compromising the integrity of the remaining coronal tooth structure that makes

up the preparation. While this problem may not be significant in the case of a single crown, the dentist is typically presented with cases that are much more extensive and complicated.

If the endodontics is attempted by conventional means, that is, through the existing restoration, the risk is high that the restoration will have to be replaced. In complicated fixed prosthodontic restorations, this may dictate the replacement of several units, or even an entire arch. Sometimes the situation is complicated by a precision or semiprecision attachment on the involved unit, which virtually assures the failure of the restoration if conventional endodontics is attempted.

Given the basic principle that endodontic surgery should be considered as an alternative to conventional endodontics in cases where it is indicated both restoratively and surgically, it is interesting to note that less than unanimous agreement exists among the endodontic community on this issue. Some endodontists are strongly opposed to performing apical surgery and retrofill procedures for the purpose of avoiding damage to an existing restoration, while others view such action as sometimes justifiable.

Leaders in the endodontic community have changed their positions on this issue over the years. For example, in his 1965 endodontics textbook Ingle listed porcelain jacket crowns, fixed bridge abutments, and dowel cores, as indications for endodontic surgery and retrofilling of teeth.[8] He believed they could preclude a conventional procedure and so were indications for retrofilling. However, in the latest edition of the same textbook, Ingle indicates that several situations, namely the first two of those above, including fixed bridge abutments and porcelain jacket crowns, previously included as indications for surgery, are now put in the nonsurgical category. He now advocates that porcelain jacket crowns and fixed bridge retainers do not preclude making access through the existing restoration and are not justifications for retrofill procedures. But he concludes these recom-

mendations with the comment that the patient should be forewarned that the crown might fracture and need replacement following root canal therapy, and that some dentists still prefer to retrofill teeth with precision attachments or crowns supporting partial denture rests.[9]

The dentist, however, must ultimately decide how the patient is to be treated, within the dictates of accepted practice in the various specialty areas. The goal is to save as much of the patient's dentition as possible for as long a time as possible, and in as good a state of health as possible.

There is no real argument over treatment indicated when a dowel core is present, particularly a cast dowel as opposed to a premade one. The choice of treatment is usually between a retrofill and extraction (Fig. 5-27).

If a tooth with a cast dowel core needs treatment for a periapical lesion, surgery may be indicated, even when the final restoration has not been cemented. The alternative will usually be extraction. Sometimes the tooth may be a critical abutment for the final restoration. For example, if the first premolar is extracted, there would no longer be any possibility of a fixed bridge. Instead, a removable partial denture would be required (Fig. 5-28). In rare cases the tooth in question may have been filled with the split silver point technique (Fig. 5-29). There is little chance, even with the use of newer methods involving ultrasonic vibration, of successfully removing most of these points because they are too small and inaccessible.

In other types of restorations such as the ones mentioned, it is ultimately the dentist who must make the final treatment decision. If the patient and the dentist feel strongly that an extensive, complex restoration would be at risk if access were attempted using the coronal approach, and if a retrofill is possible, it is in the patient's best interest to be referred to an endodontist who ascribes to a similar philosophy.

The endodontist's experience and specialized training legitimizes his or her evaluation of the need for retrofill. If the procedure is contraindicated for a case other avenues can be explored.

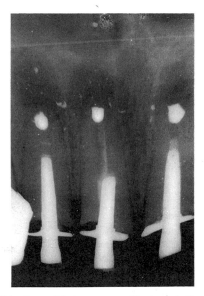

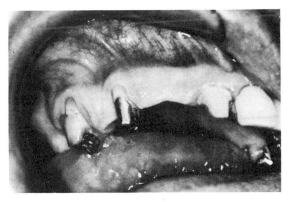

Fig. 5-28   Case involving a dowel core in the critical premolar abutment for a multiple-unit bridge.

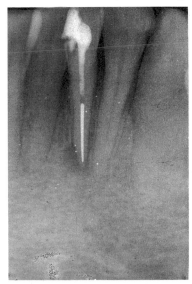

Fig. 5-27   Retrofills in a case with dowels that could not be removed without risking fracture of the root.

In such cases, other possible modes of treatment include:

1. In the case of a cast dowel, it is sometimes possible to remove the dowel by use of a high-speed handpiece. More often than not, this will be unsuccessful.
2. Ultrasonic vibration is showing some promise, but cannot be relied upon yet.
3. On occasion, a silver point can be removed using files or broaches.
4. Obviously, one alternative is to extract the tooth.

One of the primary contraindications for the surgical approach is a poor crown-to-root ratio. Ante's law states: "The total periodontal membrane area of the abutment teeth should equal or exceed that of the teeth to be replaced."[10] The radiograph in Fig. 5-30 shows that if a surgical approach were to be attempted on the premolar if it needed endodontic treatment, the result would be an even further compromised crown-to-root ratio. In such a case it is better to remove the bridge, perform conventional endodontic therapy, and construct a new bridge (Fig. 5-30).

To patients and general dentists, it might

Fig. 5-29   Split silver point, removal of which usually is not possible.

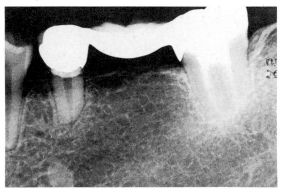

Fig. 5-30   This premolar bridge abutment would not be indicated for surgery were endodontic treatment needed, because of the poor crown-to-root ratio.

seem unjustified to risk losing retention on a ten-unit porcelain-fused-to-metal fixed bridge or a difficult-to-replace precision partial denture just because the endodontic specialist does not believe in retrofilling.

Besides the crown-to-root ratio problem, some of the following may result:

1. Surgical access may be contraindicated anatomically, such as by proximity to the maxillary sinus.
2. The patient may be a poor medical risk.
3. Periodontal disease may have changed the

clinical picture since the time the restoration was originally placed, making the surgical endodontic approach less successful than the conventional one.

The objective is not necessarily to implement the most conservative endodontic approach possible if it endangers the dentition. One text devoted entirely to endodontic surgery does not mention existing restorations as an indication for surgery.[11] Yet, from a financial and long-term health standpoint, such a restoration might justify endodontic surgery.

References

1. Kerekes, K., and Tronstad, L. Long-term results of endodontic treatment performed with a standardized technique. J. Endo. 5:8, 1979.
2. Morse, D.R., et al. A radiographic evaluation of the periapical status of teeth treated by gutta-percha-eucapercha endodontic method: A one year follow-up study of 458 root canals. Part III. Oral Surg. 56:190, 1983.
3. Levin, H.J. Access cavities. D. Clin. N. Am. 11:701–710, 1967.
4. Ingle, J.I. Endodontics. Philadelphia: Lea & Febiger, 1985.
5. Sommer, R.F., et al. Clinical Endodontics. Philadelphia and London: W.B. Saunders Co., 1956.
6. Standlee, J.P., et al. Analysis of stress distribution by endodontic posts. Oral Surg. 33:952, 1972.
7. Caputo, A.A., and Standlee, J.P. Pins and posts—Why, when, and how. D. Clin. N. Am. 20:299, 1976.
8. Ingle, J.I. Endodontics. Philadelphia: Lea & Febiger, 1965.
9. Ingle, J.I. Endodontics. Philadelphia: Lea & Febiger, 1985, p. 625.
10. Ante, I.H. The fundamental principles of abutments. Mich. Dent. Soc. Bull. 8:14, 1926.
11. Arens, D.E., et al. Endodontic Surgery. Philadelphia: Harper & Row Publ. Inc., 1981.

Additional reading

Armstrong, R.L., et al. Endodontics and the overdenture. J. Mass. Dent. Soc. 26:240–243, 1977.
Barnes, I.E. Surgical endodontics. Introduction, principles and indications. Dent. Update, 8:89–92, 95–99, 1981.
Bergenholtz, G., et al. Retreatment of endodontic fillings.

Scand. J. Dent. Res. 87:217–224, 1979.
Fors, U.G.H., and Berg, J.O. A method for the removal of broken endodontic instruments from root canals. J. Endo. 9:156–159, 1983.
Frank, A.L. Improvement of the crown-root ratio by endodontic-endosseous implants. J. Am. Dent. Assoc. 74:451, 1967.
Gaffney, J.L., et al. Expanded use of the ultrasonic scaler. J. Endo. 7:228–229, 1981.
Luebke, R.G., et al. Indications and contraindications for endodontic surgery. Oral Surg. 18:97–113, 1964.
Marotta, J.D. A prepared opening into the pulp chamber (letter). J. Prosthet. Dent. 51:135, 1984.
Mills, J.C. A study of the relationship between the endodontist and the general dentist. J. Endo. 10:110–114, 1984.
Pulver, W., et al. The first step to endodontic success: The access cavity. Ont. Dent. 53:11–13, 1976.
Rosen, H. Operative procedures on mutilated endodontically treated teeth. J. Prosthet. Dent. 11:973–986, 1961.
Rud, J., and Andreasen, J.O. Operative procedures in periapical surgery with contemporaneous root filling. Int. J. Oral Surg. 1:297–310, 1972.
Rud, J., et al. A follow-up study of 1000 cases treated by endodontic surgery. Int. J. Oral Surg. 1:215–228, 1972.
Schilder, H. Filling root canals in three dimensions. D. Clin. N. Am. 11:723–729, 1967.
Shillingburg, H.T., and Kessler, J.C. Restoration of the Endodontically Treated Tooth. Chicago: Quintessence Publ. Co., 1982.
Sieraski, S.M., and Zillich, R.M. Silver point retreatment: Review and case report. J. Endo. 9:35–39, 1983.
Spasser, H.F. Preventive endodontics. J. Prev. Dent. 2:(6)8–12, 1975.
Standlee, J.P., et al. Retention of endodontic dowels: Effects of cement, dowel length, diameter, and design. J. Prosthet. Dent. 39:400–405, 1978.
Waliszewski, K.J., et al. Combined endodontic and restorative treatment considerations. J. Prosthet. Dent. 40:152–156, 1978.
Weisman, M.I. The removal of difficult silver cones. J. Endo. 9:210–229, 1983.

Chapter 6

Marginal Defects and Perforations in Crowns

When a dentist sees a new patient or one on recall, he or she must carefully check the margins of all crowns and bridges for caries, verify that abutments of any fixed bridges are securely cemented, and complete a thorough examination. By faithfully doing this, major difficulties can potentially be prevented.

Carious margins

If caries is detected at a crown margin, or erosion at a margin has caused an opening, the usual procedure is to remove the old crown, reprepare the tooth, and make a new crown. However, on occasion it may be desirable to try saving the existing crown if:

1. The crown is part of a more extensive restoration such as a retainer for a fixed bridge or a removable partial denture. Remaking the crown would require a procedure more extensive than that used for a single crown.
2. Esthetically, the existing crown is so well made that matching it would be difficult.
3. It may be desirable to use the existing crown as a long-term temporary. A patient may find that a new crown and other required treatments are not currently affordable, even though they may be covered by dental insurance or other third-party carriers. There are usually limitations and restrictions associated with dental insurance, such as annual

maximums, which can easily be exceeded when extensive restorative treatment is necessary. One solution is treatment planning that considers the patient's financial constraints and insurance benefits/limitations. By doing this, the dentist provides a great service to patients and is able to build a practice.

Whenever an extensive delay in treatment is anticipated, caries should be treated as a temporary measure to prevent further destruction of tooth structure.

Although the most common area for carious lesions is around margins in Class V areas (Fig. 6-1), they can also occur around margins of partial veneer crowns. Caries can occur at a margin—even if the margin was originally closed completely.[1] Usually, caries occurs because the original crown had an improper fit for one or more of the following reasons:

1. Imprecise marginal definition in the preparation
2. Poor impression technique
3. Mishandling of materials
4. Laboratory error
5. Incomplete seating

These are mostly a result of operator error. Even in the case of laboratory error, the dentist should not accept a defective crown from the laboratory. In most cases, defective margins require a remake of the crown. For example, a

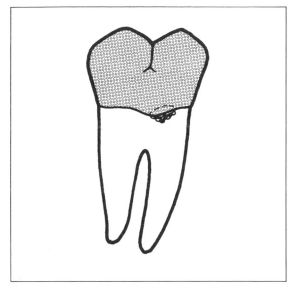

Fig. 6-1 Typical example of caries at the gingival margin extending occlusally under the crown.

crown with caries at a margin caused by incomplete seating of the casting will have other openings. In such cases this procedure is used only as a stopgap until the restoration can be replaced.

When a crown with open margins caused by incomplete seating was originally placed, the open areas were filled with cement (Fig. 6-2). Over time, the cement was dissolved by oral fluids and openings developed, resulting in caries formation in susceptible individuals (Figs. 6-3 and 6-4). The caries may be limited to the marginal area, or extend to the point of pulpal involvement. Where decay is extensive a complete remake is needed.

Dentists have often removed an existing crown with open margins and not found caries underneath it. Sometimes the crowns had been in that condition for years and the underlying teeth had not decayed, probably because that particular tooth or patient was resistant to decay. However, the absence of decay in one instance of an open margin is no justification for cementing a crown with a known open margin. A conscientious dentist will make every effort to do quality work and will not knowingly deliver defective restorations. Because caries did not

occur in one patient does not mean it will not occur in another patient or in the same patient in the future.

Marginal caries can also be brought on by an inability to clean margins because of overcontoured dental restorations, or the failure of patients to keep their teeth and gingiva plaque-free.

Gingival recession can cause previously subgingival margins to become supragingival, and occasionally the exposure of cementum can lead to caries in these areas. Also, areas of erosion or abrasion sometimes develop near exposed margins. In most of these instances, however, the area is clean and hard, and shows no evidence of caries. As long as the margins are closed, treatment is usually not needed as a result of erosion or abrasion. This can occur over a period of time due to gingival recession or can occur after periodontal surgery. Sometimes a simple Class V restoration is sufficient treatment while at other times the caries is so extensive that a conservative approach is impossible.

Perforated crowns

The second area where caries occur in relation to existing crowns is on the occlusal surface after a perforation of the crown (Figs. 6-5a and b). Perforation can be the result of normal wear of the opposing dentition, bruxism, or a thin initial crown. The latter is usually caused by inadequate occlusal reduction in the preparation. Once the metal has been worn through, caries can occur on occlusal surfaces in the same ways they occur in areas around marginal openings.

Some basic conditions need to be met when deciding to save the crown on a short- or long-term basis:

1. The operator must have clear access to all anticipated cavosurface margins. In Class V areas, the gingiva must be completely out of the way. When the caries extends interprox-

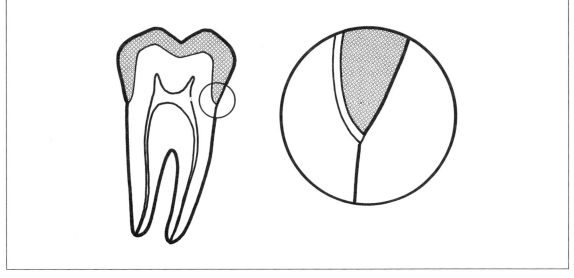

Fig. 6-2 Circled area shows the crown-to-tooth junction of an incompletely seated crown with cement present.

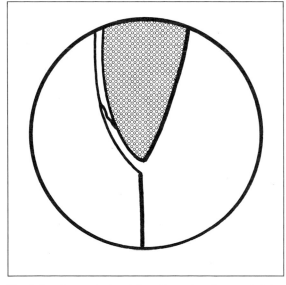

Fig. 6-3 Crown-to-tooth junction of an incompletely seated crown with cement washed out.

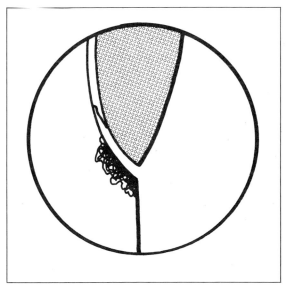

Fig. 6-4 Crown-to-tooth junction of an incompletely seated crown with development of caries.

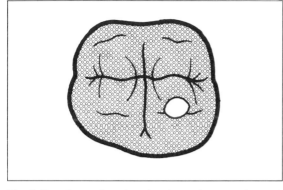

Fig. 6-5a Area of perforation in occlusal surface of gold crown.

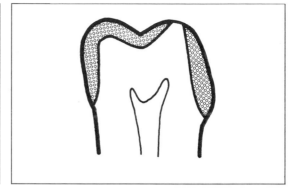

Fig. 6-5b Cross-section of perforation on occlusal surface of gold crown resulting from inadequate occlusal reduction.

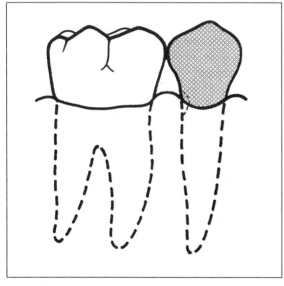

Fig. 6-6 Interproximal marginal caries in an inaccessible area on the distal surface of the premolar.

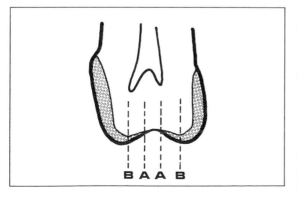

imally, particularly on the distal and lingual surfaces, access can be so difficult as to preclude treatment (Fig. 6-6). Whenever any cavosurface margin is inaccessible, this procedure should not be attempted. Methods for gaining complete access will be discussed later in this chapter.

2. The operator must have clear visual access to all internal areas of the preparation, either directly, or indirectly with a mirror, to verify the removal of all carious lesions. Inaccessibility causes problems in the interproximal areas, or where caries spread laterally or occlusally under the margin of the crown. If access cannot be gained, the crown must be removed and redone with all other considerations aside except for the short-term control of caries.

3. The operator must be able to keep the working area dry and free of moisture contamination. Specific methods for moisture control are detailed later in this chapter.

4. The caries cannot be so extensive as to have weakened the tooth and compromised resistance or retention.

5. The area around an occlusal perforation is likely to be thin (Fig. 6-7). The cavity prepara-

Fig. 6-7 Cross-section of crown with occlusal perforation. (*A—A*) shows the area of actual perforation. (*A—B*) shows the thin area around the perforation.

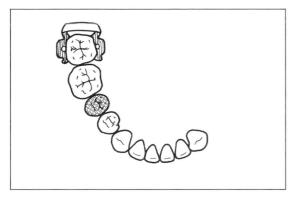

Fig. 6-8 Rubber dam in place.

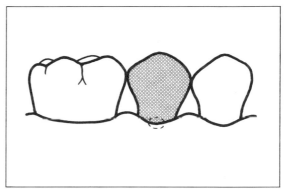

Fig. 6-9 Typical location of Class V caries at gold-to-tooth junction.

tion must be enlarged to get to an area where the remaining casting is sufficiently thick to prevent further perforation. If adequate thickness cannot be obtained, a new crown must be made after sufficient occlusal reduction.

Field isolation and moisture control

After the preceding criteria are met, access and moisture control become important considerations. The following techniques will help gain access and control moisture.

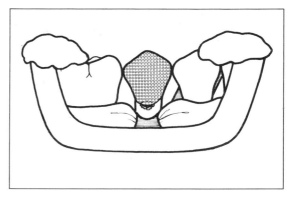

Fig. 6-10 Class V subgingival caries at gold-to-tooth junction with rubber dam and no. 212 clamp in place. All areas of caries are well-exposed.

Method: Rubber dam

Step 1

A rubber dam is usually the best method for moisture control and gaining accessibility to most areas of the mouth. Normal placement of a rubber dam often provides sufficient gingival retraction. Isolation includes two teeth distal to the one being treated, when possible, and extends to the midline or canine on the opposite side of the mouth to provide a clear, dry, working field (Fig. 6-8).

In other cases the rubber dam will not sufficiently retract the gingiva (Fig. 6-9). Adequate retraction can often be accomplished in these

cases by using a no. 212 rubber dam clamp (Fig. 6-10), or one similarly designed. This clamp can expose 2 to 3 mm of additional tooth structure and can be the difference between success and failure.

Step 2

When using a no. 212 rubber dam clamp, the hole for the clamp should be placed 1 to 2 mm facially to what would be the normal position of the tooth (Fig. 6-11).

Sometimes when using a no. 212 rubber dam clamp to retract the gingiva, it will be necessary to place two relieving incisions 2 or 3 mm long to avoid tearing the gingiva (Fig. 6-12). Make

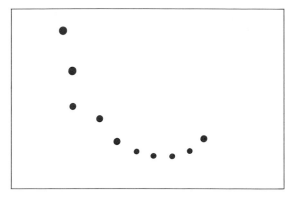

Fig. 6-11 Rubber dam with modification of position of holes for teeth.

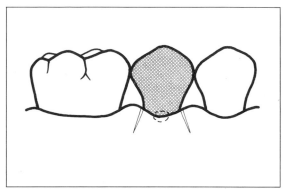

Fig. 6-12 Two relieving incisions in gingiva allowing for gingival retraction.

sharp, clean incisions to allow the gingiva to heal quickly with little or no recession.[2] If the gingiva tears, which could occur if the incisions are not made, healing is much slower and recession is more frequent. It is normally unnecessary to suture these incisions.

Method: Surgical flap

Occasionally, it is necessary to reflect a flap to gain adequate access, and even to reduce some crestal bone in rare cases. It is essential to thoroughly clean the area of any remaining filling material or other debris before suturing it closed. This procedure would normally be accomplished in conjunction with a periodontist. A periodontal dressing is often advised in these cases. While these procedures may seem drastic, if an open or inadequate margin is left because of poor access, further decay will ensue and may cause tooth loss.

Method: Electrosurgery

Another method for gaining adequate access and moisture control in Class V areas is electrosurgery. The technique is effective where areas of caries are small or extend subgingivally a short distance. It is not recommended as a method of access and moisture control when there is inadequate attached gingiva, accute inflammation, or extensive subgingival caries.

Electrosurgery may also be used in posterior areas when a rubber dam clamp placement will interfere with adequate access to the carious area.

Method: Gingival retraction cord

Where subgingival caries is minimal, gingival retraction cord can provide adequate access to all margins, and control moisture. The smallest cord with the mildest medication for adequate retraction is recommended. It is often possible to use a gingival retraction cord without drugs, since temporary displacement of the tissue is all that is necessary. Leaving a cord impregnated with epinephrine or alum in the crevice for the period required by this procedure can damage tissue. The objective is to attain the maximum retraction with minimal tissue damage.

If using retraction cord, care must be taken not to tear the gingiva when packing it. In addition, when cord is too deeply packed or too large, circulation to the tissue can be cut off, followed by sloughing off of this tissue and resulting in gingival recession. Use of epinephrine cord is not recommended because it will aggravate the problem. After placing the retraction cord so that the area of the eventual margins of the preparation is exposed, leave the cord in place while completing the preparation. If the cord is still dry, it can remain while the restorative material is placed, but if the cord is saturated, replace it and then place the filling material.

Method: Silk suture material

Use 000 silk suture material the same way retraction cord is used to provide limited retraction and moisture control. This material has two important features: (1) There are no drugs in this material to cause adverse gingival or systemic reactions, and (2) It does not absorb tissue fluids and does not become saturated. However, silk does not provide as much retraction or moisture control as cord, so it should only be used when the need for retraction and moisture control is minimal.

Summary of moisture control

Use the simplest and quickest method for gaining access and controlling moisture. Good clinical judgment is essential when deciding which method to use. Sometimes, a combination of the preceding techniques will enable all caries to be removed and the teeth restored to proper contours and function. A rubber dam with or without a flap usually provides the best access and moisture control for the longest period. Its main drawback is the amount of time involved for placement. Cord and/or electrosurgery is quick and simple but does not provide as much access or moisture control for as long a time as rubber dam. More recession is associated with the use of cord or electrosurgery, but tissue damage can occur with any method if the tissue is not properly handled.

Restoration of Class V defects in existing restorations

Method

Step 1

Once the lesion has been isolated, remove the caries and create sufficient retention for the restoration. The size and shape of the cavity preparation will be dictated almost completely by the extent of the caries (Figs. 6-13a and b). The preparation should have rounded external angles. Sharp cavosurface angles make it more difficult to properly condense silver amalgam, and lead to an excess concentration of mercury at these points. It may be necessary to remove some of the margin area of the crown with the bur to ascertain that all caries that extends along the crown to tooth interface is removed (Fig. 6-14). When the existing restoration is a porcelain-to-metal crown, the dentist must not weaken the existing porcelain by cutting into it. When the caries extends too far under a porcelain-to-metal crown, rule out this procedure and make a new crown.

Step 2

After removing all caries, remove weakened or unsupported tooth structure, and achieve retention by undercutting the occlusal and gingival margins by .5 to 1.0 mm. Adequately base deep areas to protect the pulpal tissues (Fig. 6-15).

Step 3

The final restoration will be either amalgam, composite, or gold foil. Amalgam has been shown to be an adequate filling material around gold crowns in terms of microleakage. Both high-copper and low-copper hand-condensed alloys used according to manufacturer's instructions, and carved to proper contours, have been shown to be successful when placed in contact with gold crowns.[3] In areas susceptible to mois-

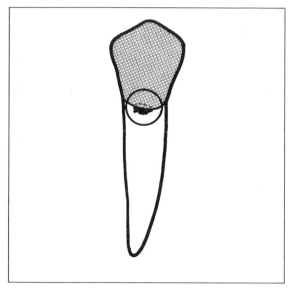

Fig. 6-13a Class V caries at the gold-to-tooth junction.

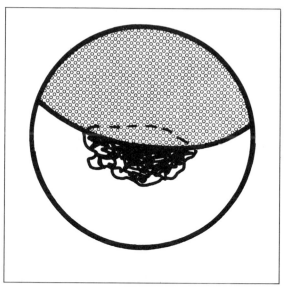

Fig. 6-13b Close up of lesion showing extension of caries occlusally under crown.

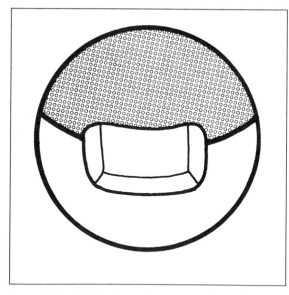

Fig. 6-14 Finished cavity preparation showing rounded external-line angles and extension occlusally into the gold crown.

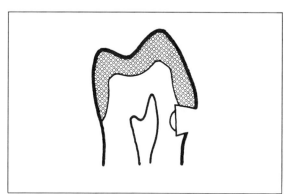

Fig. 6-15 Cross-section of cavity preparation showing undercuts, extension into gold crown, and placement of base, if necessary.

ture contamination, zinc-free amalgam is recommended. Burnishing the amalgam after the initial set and/or polishing the amalgam after final set provides a surface that is smooth, compatible with the gingiva, less susceptible to plaque buildup, easier to keep clean, and longer-lasting than unpolished amalgam.

The cavity may be restored with light-cured composite in areas of the mouth where esthetics is critical. A microfill composite is recommended because it can be polished to a higher degree.

When using composite, it is essential to place adequate occlusal and gingival retention grooves to reduce marginal microleakage. Composites will usually not last as long as amalgams in these areas because of microleakage. However, in anterior areas of the mouth where amalgam is esthetically unacceptable, composite material is preferable.

A third restorative material is gold foil. Gold foil is expensive for the patient and very technique-sensitive; any moisture contamination will cause failure. Therefore, a rubber dam is essential, and unless a dentist has acquired an adeptness with gold foil through regular use, the material is not recommended.

Restoration of Class I defects in existing restorations

Seeing a patient with a crown perforated on the occlusal surface is not uncommon. The following are some of the causes of this defect:

1. Insufficient occlusal clearance initially causes a perforation after a moderate amount of wear or occlusal adjustment. This is by far the most common cause of the problem.
2. A defect in the casting, which after a time is broken through by occlusal forces or is actually ground through during the insertion procedure. This defect is usually caused by a "suck-back porosity" during the casting process.

The area around the perforation is likely to be thin. It must be possible to make a preparation large enough to reach to an area where the remaining casting is sufficiently thick to prevent further perforation and protect the integrity of the casting. If this is impossible, or if doing so causes a Class I preparation that is too large, then a new crown must be made after removing the old one and attaining adequate occlusal reduction.

There are several methods and materials for correcting an occlusal perforation when the aforementioned requirements have been satisfied. Among them are amalgam or direct gold restoration, and cast gold inlay.

Method: Amalgam or direct gold restoration

Step 1

Isolate the area and control moisture as you would in any direct filling procedure done with these materials.

Step 2

Enlarge the opening at the site of the perforation until the minimum thickness of the casting as seen on the axial walls of the preparation is at least .50 mm (Fig. 6-16). If this creates an excessively large opening, make a new crown regardless of any other considerations. Any enlargement of more than 25% of the occlusal table should be considered excessive (Fig. 6-17).

Step 3

After attaining adequate thickness of the remaining casting on the axial walls of the preparation, it is necessary to create an adequate depth. This should amount to 1.5 mm or more and the axial walls should be slightly undercut. With a direct gold filling, this depth might need to be increased to attain adequate length of dentin walls below the casting for proper

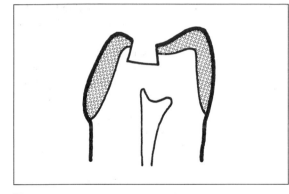

Fig. 6-16 Direct-filling preparation into gold crown with slightly undercut walls. Gold is .5 mm thick and preparation floor is in solid tooth structure or buildup.

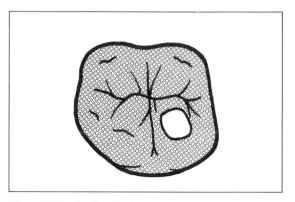

Fig. 6-17 Occlusal view of preparation into gold crown. Outline is determined by thickness of gold casting.

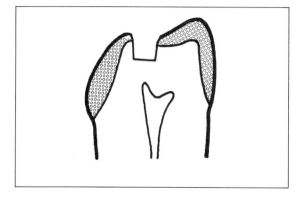

Fig. 6-18 Inlay preparation in gold crown. Preparation is deeper than one for direct filling, with flared walls and slight bevel at occlusal finish lines.

elasticity which is essential when using this material. For this step, use an inverted cone bur, usually a no. 34. The floor of this preparation must be in dentin or a solid buildup material such as amalgam or composite, not just cement, so that resistance to apical displacement in occlusion can be realized (Fig. 6-16).

Step 4

Place the amalgam or gold foil, burnish margins, remove the rubber dam or other isolation devices and adjust the occlusion.

Method: Cast gold inlay

Step 1

Gain adequate isolation of the area and control moisture as you would in any cast gold preparation procedure. Normally, this will not require the rubber dam.

Step 2

Enlarge the opening at the site of the perforation, in this case developing a preparation which has flared axial walls as for any typical Class I inlay. Apply the same requirements as for the amalgam method in terms of size limitations (Fig. 6-17). However, for preparation depth, a greater depth may be needed, because an inlay derives its retention from the fit and area of cementation on the axial walls (Fig. 6-18).

Step 3

Make an impression of the preparation using the material and method of the operator's choice. An excellent procedure is the double-bite impression, in which both maxillary and mandibular quadrant cast are simultaneously generated in perfect occlusion (see chapter 9).

Step 4

Fabricate and cement the inlay.

Summary

Placing a restoration around or into an existing crown can be an acceptable procedure when the criteria of adequate access to all margins, the removal of all caries, and adequate moisture control are met. Marginal failures can be avoided by applying principles of preventative dentistry and by good initial patient care.

Careful initial preparation of teeth with emphasis on adequate reduction occlusally and axially, as well as proper marginal placement, enable the laboratory technician to fabricate a proper crown.

An accurate impression technique sometimes requires using electrosurgery and more than one impression if the first one is unsatisfactory. Use of a stereomicroscope to examine the impression for voids, missing margins, and trimming dies can be invaluable. The microscope is also helpful in waxing margins and determining that a casting properly fits the die. Proper use of the die spacer helps ensure that the crown is correctly seated. Use of topical fluoride and instruction in proper dental hygiene can reduce marginal caries, particularly after patients have had periodontal surgery.

References

1. Kantorowicz, G.F. The repair and removal of bridges. Dent. Pract. 21:341–346, 1971.
2. Wolcott, R. Operative dentistry (Unpublished syllabus). School of Dentistry, University of California at Los Angeles, 1968.
3. Fitch, D.R., et al. Amalgam repair of cast crown margins: A microleakage assessment. Gen. Dent. 328–330, 1982.

Additional reading

Mansfield, W.J. Treatment of proximal marginal caries in crowned teeth. J. Prosthet. Dent. 51:49–50, 1984.

Chapter 7

Buildups Under Existing Restorations

When a previously cemented crown loses retention or is defective, it is often desirable to save the crown as a final restoration, rather than make a new crown. The existing crown may be a good one in terms of fit, contour, and esthetics, or it may be part of a more extensive restoration such as an abutment for a fixed bridge or a removable partial denture. If it is lost, a more extensive remake is necessary, and financial considerations may make saving the existing crown desirable. In determining whether to save the crown or to make a new one, consider the following factors:

1. Marginal fit
2. Interproximal contacts—both tightness and contour
3. Occlusion
4. Axial contours
5. Esthetics
6. Structural integrity of the restoration itself
7. Retention form of the original preparation, as reflected by the internal form of the restoration

If the existing crown is inadequate in any of these areas and that deficiency cannot be overcome, then a new crown should be made, regardless of any other considerations. For example, an open interproximal contact may be corrected since the crown is out of the mouth, but an open margin will require a new crown. Also, in the case of a single unit, the cost involved in saving the old restoration should be less than that of making a new crown. However, in the case of units involved in more complex restorations, this factor may play a lesser role in the decision-making process. The tooth supporting the restoration must be free of pathology, as determined by a full oral and radiographic examination. The presence of such things as a periapical abcess or a treatable periodontal pocket does not necessarily rule out salvaging the existing crown. However, it is essential that any pathologic process be controlled or eliminated before attempting to save the existing restoration.

Attention should be paid not only to the periodontal health of the tooth in question, but also to that of other teeth in the arch that may affect the treatment plan. It is dangerous to focus undue attention on the tooth to be corrected while ignoring the effects of time and inadequate oral hygiene on other teeth. The situation may well be quite different than when this restoration was originally conceived and constructed. Periodontal or endodontic problems in surrounding teeth must also be treated if the existing restoration is to be successfully saved.

There are many methods for constructing buildups under existing crowns.[1-10] Most involve placing a quick-curing acrylic resin inside the crown and the canal, or around pins, and then placing the crown back on the tooth with the excess resin extruded between the margins of the crown and the tooth when the crown is pressed into place. Sometimes a post cemented prior to placing resin around it allows a

Table 7-1 Indications for best methods for buildups under existing crowns

Method	Indications
Pin-retained buildup	Vital tooth, intact margins, sound root structure, crown can be removed
Preformed post	Endodontically treated tooth, intact margins, sound root structure, may or may not be able to remove crown
Cast post	Endodontically treated tooth, crown can usually be removed, sound root, margins intact

one-step buildup. In others, by using a plastic pin a pattern is cast and cemented before the crown is placed. Two major difficulties make these techniques unacceptable. First, it is difficult to verify that the crown is perfectly seated when it is sufficiently filled with resin for replacing the fractured coronal portion of the tooth. Second, even if the crown is correctly seated, a film of resin of varying thicknesses at the margins will always be present.

Table 7-1 lists the techniques that eliminate these problems: pin-retained buildup, preformed post, and cast post. The method involving a cast post and core is a modification of an accepted technique.[11] The choice of technique depends on the status of the abutment tooth and the existing restoration. Table 7-1 presents the indications for each method.

Pin-retained buildup under existing restoration

A pin-retained buildup has the advantage of maintaining the vitality of the pulp. It is usually the quickest and least expensive method for saving an existing crown that has lost retention. The disadvantages of the pin-retained buildup are primarily related to retention of the pins in the tooth structure, and to the risk to the pulpal health or root perforation when pin placement is not ideal.

A pin-retained buildup can be used when part of the underlying tooth structure of a vital tooth is lost and retention of the casting has been compromised. This situation can arise when part of the tooth is fractured during removal of a temporary restoration, when the final restoration is removed during the try-in phase or after a period of temporary cementation, or when a permanently cemented crown loses retention via loss of underlying tooth structure.

Often the crown can be saved and reused if a pin-retained buildup is used in addition to the remaining sound tooth structure for adequate crown retention. Complete the endodontic therapy if the preparation needs additional retention and support from an endodontic post.

Use a pin-retained buildup only when it will provide adequate strength and retention for the crown. Explanations of the techniques involving endodontic posts will be discussed later in this chapter.

The following are two variations on these methods:

1. In the first method, the buildup material is injected through an opening in the occlusal or lingual surface of the crown after first seating the pins in the tooth.

2. In the second method, a die and a matrix made of a copper band and modeling compound are utilized. The die will usually be available if the buildup is needed prior to final cementation. If the die is not available, one may be fabricated by using the existing casting and pouring die stone inside. When the stone has set, the casting and die are separated and the die is trimmed. Use of a light coat of petroleum jelly inside the casting prior to pouring the die stone will facilitate separation after the stone has hardened.

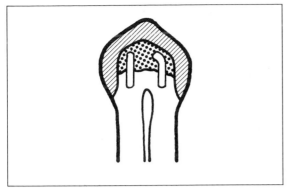

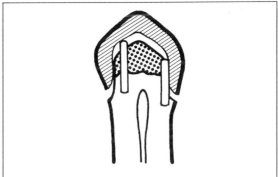

Fig. 7-1 Cross-section of a premolar with two properly placed pins retaining a buildup. Pins are within the preparation and do not interfere with seating of the crown.

Fig. 7-2 Cross-section of premolar with two improperly placed pins. Both pins are outside the area of initial preparation and prevent complete seating of the crown.

Method: Pin-retained buildup

Use this first pin-retained method when a critical part of the underlying vital tooth structure is lost and casting retention is compromised. This can occur when tooth structure is fractured during removal of a temporary restoration; during removal of the final restoration during the try-in phase or after a period of temporary cementation; or when a permanently cemented crown loses retention due to loss of underlying tooth structure. The crown can often be saved and reused when a pin-retained buildup is used in addition to the remaining sound tooth structure to provide adequate crown retention. If the preparation needs the added retention and support provided by an endodontic post, then endodontic therapy must be completed.

Step 1

Verify the reusability of the crown. All the margins must be present and the fit must meet the same criteria as if the crown were being placed for the first time. Interproximal contacts, contour, and occlusion must also be adequate. The only defect would be lack of retention.

Step 2

Place enough self-threading pins to properly retain the new buildup. Since the crown is off the tooth, this procedure is the same for building up any tooth to receive a full crown, with the following exceptions:

1. Since the form of the crown preparation has already been determined, the pins must be placed within the inner form of the existing crown so that they do not interfere with seating of the crown. The pins will usually need to be bent after placement with the correct bending tool, which is usually supplied with the pin kit (Figs. 7-1 and 7-2).

2. Some clinicians prefer to cut off excess pin length after the buildup material has set so that less stress is applied to the dentin. However, in this technique, it is essential that the pins be cut to the proper length *before* the buildup is placed, to allow the crown to be seated all the way to the margin. Wire cutters can be used after screwing the pins into the dentin, or the apical ends of the pins can be cut off prior to screwing them in. Placing grooves in the remaining dentin coronally to the margins will give added retention.

Step 3

Create a small opening in the occlusal surface of a posterior casting or the lingual surface of an anterior casting. The opening must be of ade-

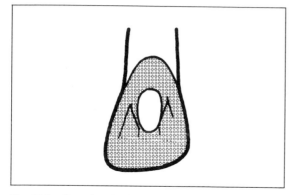

Fig. 7-3 Opening in lingual surface of a maxillary anterior crown.

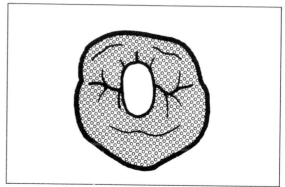

Fig. 7-4 Occlusal opening in a crown for a posterior tooth.

quate size to allow the composite buildup material to be injected through it using a composite syringe.* The hole must be oval rather than round so that air will be allowed to escape between the syringe tip and the crown when the composite is injected through the crown in a subsequent step (Figs. 7-3 and 7-4).

Step 4

Place the crown on the tooth and verify that the pins do not interefere with seating or with injecting the composite. If the pins interfere, shorten or bend them to allow the crown to seat (Figs. 7-1 and 7-2).

Step 5

Remove the crown and place calcium hydroxide over any exposed dentin close to the pulp. Lubricate the inner surface of the crown with petroleum jelly or tin-foil substitute. This step is indispensable to removing the crown after the composite has set.

Step 6

Replace the crown and stabilize it with either softened compound or acrylic resin.** Softened

compound can be adapted to the facial and lingual surfaces of the crown and the teeth mesial and distal to it. Connecting the two matrices thus generated, with some compound running over the occlusal surfaces from facial to lingual, will prevent either from detaching. The importance of this step cannot be overemphasized. It is simply not reliable to attempt to hold the crown in position with the fingers while injecting the buildup material (Figs. 7-5 and 7-6).

Acrylic resin can be used instead of compound to temporarily connect the adjacent teeth with the crown. Place the powder and liquid in separate dappen dishes, and lightly place a small brush in the powder to form a small bead of wet resin. Place this wet resin bead on one marginal ridge of the crown and one marginal ridge of the adjacent tooth, allowing the material to flow into the interproximal contact area. While the resin is setting, an assistant should hold the crown in proper position manually or with a dental instrument so that the dentist can use an explorer to verify that the casting is perfectly seated. After the resin has set, repeat this procedure on the other marginal ridge (Figs. 7-7 and 7-8).

Step 7

Verify that the seating is complete and the crown is stable. If it is not, break away the compound stabilizing matrices or resin and repeat step 6.

*CR Syringe, Centrix Inc., Stratford, Conn.
**Duralay Resin, Reliance Dental Manufacturing Co., Worth, Ill.

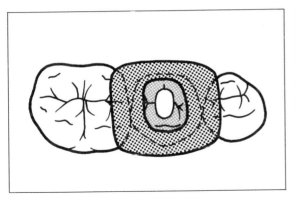

Fig. 7-5 Occlusal view of a crown over a fractured preparation being stabilized with compound.

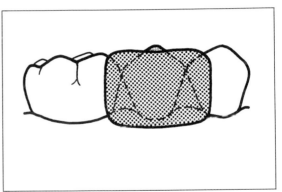

Fig. 7-6 Facial view of a crown over a fractured preparation being stabilized with compound.

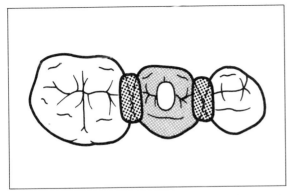

Fig. 7-7 Occlusal view of a crown over a fractured preparation being stabilized with acrylic resin.

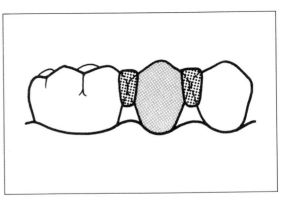

Fig. 7-8 Facial view of a crown over a fractured preparation being stabilized with acrylic resin.

Step 8

Mix equal parts base and activator of any conventional (not light-cured) crown buildup composite material. Inject it through the opening in the occlusal or lingual surface of the crown, being careful that the syringe tip does not totally occlude the opening. If it does, the following three problems may ensue:

1. The buildup material may not completely fill the inside of the crown because of air entrapment.
2. The operator will not be able to ascertain when the crown is completely filled.
3. The hydraulic pressure generated may lift the crown off the preparation slightly, allow-

ing composite to flow between the crown and the finish line of the preparation. Carefully assess this possibility before the final cementation of the crown, and if it did occur, cut away the entire new buildup, save the pins, and repeat the procedure. There must be intimate contact between the margin of the crown and the finish line of the tooth. Any buildup material allowed to extrude between the margin of the crown and the finish line of the tooth will directly cause incomplete seating of the crown.

Eliminate these problems by making the opening oval, preventing the round syringe tip from occluding it. Allow buildup material to set completely. Use of a coloring agent in the com-

133

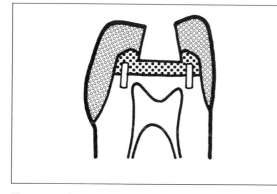

Fig. 7-9 Cross-section of a pin-retained buildup under a crown with preparation for direct filling material. Walls are slightly undercut.

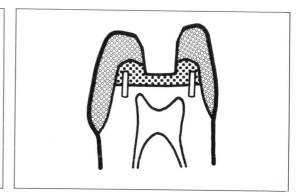

Fig. 7-10 Cross-section of pin-retained buildup under a crown with preparation for cast gold inlay. Note slightly flared walls and bevelled finish lines.

posite such as black or deep purple will facilitate the examination of the final buildup after removing the crown to absolutely ensure that none of the buildup material has extruded between the crown and the tooth at the finish line. Add a coloring agent by rubbing a pencil of the desired color on the mixing pad before mixing the composite. Mix the composite over the colored part of the pad to add color to the mix. Precolored buildup material is also available from many manufacturers of composite materials.

Step 9

Remove the crown and inspect the buildup for defects such as voids or buildup material on a finish line. Small voids may be ignored or filled in with additional buildup material as long as there is adequate retention. However, any buildup material on the finish line of the tooth will necessitate removing and replacing the entire new buildup. Simply removing the material from the offending area would cause an open margin, since the remaining new buildup will position the crown so that removing the material on a finish line will prevent the crown from seating any further. It will often be necessary to drill out the buildup material that set in the access opening before removing the crown. If difficulty is encountered in removing the crown from the

new buildup, use a Richwill crown remover according to the method outlined in chapter 2.

Step 10

Place the crown onto the new buildup and verify the marginal fit. The rest of the procedure is similar to seating any crown.

Step 11

Remove the crown and clean off any debris, such as the separating medium, with an appropriate solvent. Cement the crown as with any other restoration. The crown will probably be easier to seat completely because it is vented. Special treatment of the opening on a porcelain occlusal surface will be discussed in the next step.

Step 12

Close the access opening in the occlusal surface by one of the following means:

1. If the crown is gold, or porcelain-fused-to-metal with the access through the metal portion, make a Class I preparation by removing all cement to the level of the buildup material. Place either an amalgam or inlay restoration to fill the defect (Figs. 7-9 and 7-10). Resto-

rations involving endodontically treated teeth are discussed in full in chapter 5.

2. If the crown is porcelain-fused-to-metal with access through the porcelain, fill the defect with composite for esthetic purposes. The porcelain part of the preparation should be slightly flared as for the inlay preparation. It is neither advisable nor necessary to undercut this part of the preparation as for an amalgam or foil, since this would weaken the remaining porcelain. A slight undercut between the metal and the buildup material will give some mechanical retention. The key to this procedure is a silane bonding material which will enable the composite to join with the remaining porcelain to make a tight, strong seal. A light-cured composite is recommended for the filling material because of its superior properties and ease of use. Chapters 3 and 5 detail this technique for closing access openings in crowns.

3. Baking porcelain across the defect in the porcelain area of porcelain-fused-to-metal crowns can occasionally be done to close the defect. Unlike the first two methods, this third method requires a laboratory procedure and a subsequent dental appointment. In many cases, this will not be the method of choice because of the difficulties of doing so on a crown that has been in the mouth for a long time. Both contamination of the restoration and gassing often present complications when a crown baked by another laboratory is refired. Unknown factors in the initial construction of the crown might predispose it to liberation of gas under the porcelain on subsequent refiring. This can be compounded if the previous dentist or laboratory technician used a different alloy or porcelain. Because of these risks, a porcelain-fused-to-metal crown should be refired only when the crown was designed and constructed by the present dentist and laboratory using the same materials and techniques.

If the dentist decides to bake porcelain over the defect, there are two methods: bake the defect over with new porcelain, or remove all the porcelain and bake new porcelain on the present coping. The latter method obviates the need for a new impression with its attendant gingival retraction, which is an advantage in some cases. If the defect is simply to be filled, make a transfer cast and bake new porcelain with a platinum foil matrix.

A transfer cast is also used if all the porcelain is to be replaced, with the additional step of making a cameo model of the overall contour of the existing crown before stripping off the old porcelain. It would also be necessary in this case to supply the technician with a new shade, though in the previous situation duplicating the shade of the remaining porcelain is sufficient.

Method: Pin-retained buildup

This method is a modification of one initially advocated by Brady.[12] The goal is the same as for the first method: a crown that fits the original prepared tooth finish line, and meets the same criteria as that of the original seating.

The existing inner form of the crown is used to develop the form of the buildup.

Step 1

Verify the fit of the crown to the remaining tooth structure; all margins must be present and closed. Adjust occlusal and interproximal contacts if necessary to meet accepted criteria, and verify that 2 mm of sound tooth structure exist coronally to the finish line.

Step 2

Prepare a matrix by selecting a copper band that fits the original die, or a die made from the casting (Fig. 7-11). If die spacer was used on the original die, carefully remove this with solvent.

Adapt the band to the die and make a small opening in the middle of the facial and lingual surfaces of the band (Fig. 7-12). Place some softened, low-temperature modeling compound inside the copper band and make an impression of the die. Chill the die and compound in cold water and then carefully separate the impres-

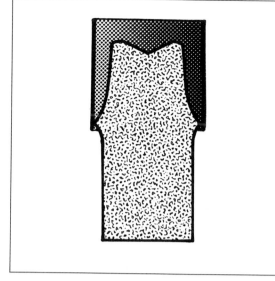

Fig. 7-11 Cross-section of stone die with adapted copper band filled with compound.

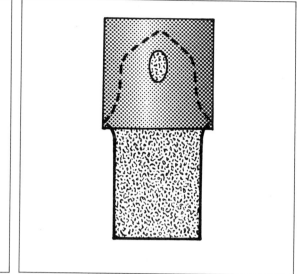

Fig. 7-12 Facial view of copper band on die with opening to allow for escape of composite. A similar opening is also on lingual surface of copper band.

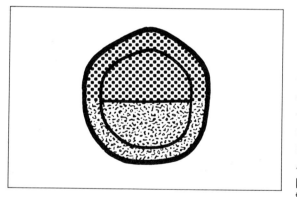

Fig. 7-13 Occlusal view of copper band and compound on die with part of compound cut away for injection of composite buildup material.

sion and the die when it has set. Remove the compound from the two vent holes and half of the occlusal surface with a scalpel blade (Fig. 7-13). Reseat the matrix on the die and verify its fit. Do the same in the mouth. The matrix should be stable, and should not bind interproximally, seating all the way to the finish lines without impinging on the gingival tissue.

Step 3

Place the appropriate number of coatings of die spacer recommended by the manufacturer of the material used on the inside of the matrix. This is tantamount to using the die spacer on the die initially, if the steps for developing the wax pattern were being followed in the usual manner. Place enough self-threading pins in the remaining tooth structure to retain a buildup. Additional retention may also be obtained by placing grooves in the remaining dentin with a tapered fissure bur such as a number 169L.

Step 4

Replace the crown on the tooth and verify that the pins do not interfere with its seating. If they do, shorten or bend them to allow the crown to seat completely to the finish lines (Figs. 7-1 and 7-2). Remove the crown and place a calcium hydroxide base such as Dycal* over any dentin close to the pulp.

*L. D. Caulk Co., Milford, Del.

Step 5

Retract the gingival tissue with cord if necessary and place the copper band matrix on the tooth. Check again for complete seating and stability. Stabilize the matrix with compound attached to the teeth mesially and distally (Fig. 7-14).

Step 6

Mix equal parts of base and catalyst of any conventional composite and use a composite syringe to inject through the opening of the matrix around the pins until the composite comes out the facial, lingual, and occlusal openings. Use a contrasting colored material to distinguish between tooth structure and buildup material. Allow the composite to set.

Step 7

Remove the matrix by cutting the copper band on the facial with a bur and peeling it away. Particular care must be taken that the finish line remains intact. Inspect the buildup for flash or voids. Any composite on the finish line of the preparation requires removing entirely the new buildup and repeating the procedure. Remove the excess composite on the occlusal which flowed out of the opening as well as that which came out of the facial and lingual relief holes.

Step 8

Seat the crown on the new buildup and verify marginal fit and stability. A silicone wash will be helpful in identifying the cause of an imperfect fit. Refer to chapter 9 for details of this procedure.

Step 9

Cement the crown in the usual manner. Since this method does not involve placing an opening in the crown, there is no need to correct the crown. However, the quality of fit to the new buildup is dependent on how well the matrix fits

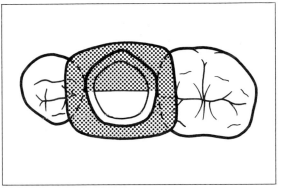

Fig. 7-14 Copper band and compound over a fractured, prepared tooth stabilized with compound that is adapted to the adjacent teeth.

the die. Any voids or looseness of the compound to the die will cause a larger buildup and subsequent tightness of the casting to the tooth at that specific point. These potential difficulties may be tolerated in the interest of avoiding problems caused by placing a hole in the occlusal surface of the crown. While a skilled dentist should be able to handle this method, it is somewhat more technique-sensitive than the one which does not involve a die and impression.

Buildups involving the pulp canal

When a crown loses retention, and the existing casting is to be reused, if the buildup will require using the canal for either a cast dowel and core, or a preformed post, endodontic therapy will need to be completed if not previously done. The endodontic result must have a good seal at the apex, good condensation, and must be of gutta-percha rather than silver point technique. If the tooth has a silver point filling, remove it, if possible, and place a proper gutta-percha filling.

Inform the patient at the outset that attempting to remove the silver point risks the loss of the remaining root. Ascertain that the tooth and surrounding tissues are free of pathology, as determined by oral and radiographic examination. If pathology exists, treat it prior to building up the tooth.

Table 7-2 Preformed post and core vs. cast post and core

Indications	Contraindications
Preformed post and core	
1. Anterior teeth when significant tooth structure remains	1. Anterior teeth when most coronal tooth is missing
2. Posterior teeth when more than one canal may be utilized for posts	2. Oval-shaped canals that would require a very large post space to create a round preparation in which to fit the preformed post
3. Post that is retentive and fitting snugly without rocking	3. A canal that is larger than the preformed posts
4. Short roots	
Cast post and core	
1. Anterior teeth when most coronal tooth is missing	1. Multirooted teeth when more than one canal must be used for retention
2. Large or oval-shaped canals	

In deciding whether to use a cast dowel and core or a preformed post and core, consider several factors because there are indications and contraindications for each (see Table 7-2).

Preformed post and core

Use this technique whenever a preformed post and buildup is the chosen treatment, provided all margins are present and intact and that all other criteria for an acceptable restoration are satisfied, except for retention. A modification of this technique may also be used after endodontic therapy is performed through the occlusal or lingual of a previously cemented crown or bridge to prevent fracture of the remaining tooth. In such a case the casting would not have lost retention, but the loss of tooth structure is a concern as a result of making the access opening. The cemented post and buildup replace the tooth structure lost in creating the access opening.

Method: Crowns with lost retention

Step 1. Remove caries and unsupported weakened tooth structure. Try-in the crown and verify that all margins are present and closed, and that all other criteria are met for seating a crown.

Step 2. Determine which canal or canals to use for the preformed post, such as a Parapost.* Use the largest, more nearly straight canal as a first choice. However, the chosen canal must enable the post to be properly positioned in the coronal area to retain the buildup material and simultaneously remain within the confines of the proposed preparation. More than one canal may be used in a multirooted tooth, or a self-threading pin may be added for rotation resistance or auxiliary retention (Figs. 7-15 and 7-16).

*Whaledent International, New York, N.Y.

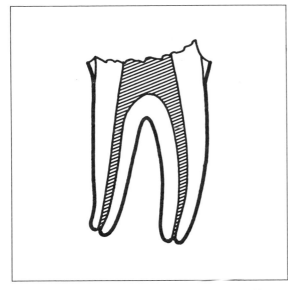

Fig. 7-15 Cross-section of fractured mandibular molar. Canals have been filled with gutta-percha. Fracture is coronal to finish line in all areas.

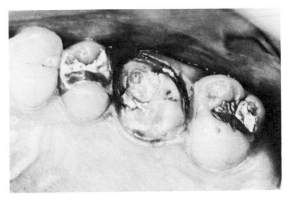

Fig. 7-16 Maxillary molar which fractured after previous crown cementation. Finish lines are all present but preparation is not retentive.

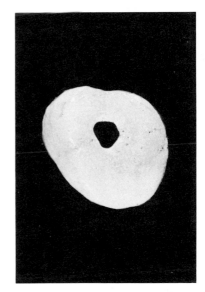

Fig. 7-17 Opening on occlusal surface of previously cemented maxillary molar crown that has lost retention because of preparation fracture.

Step 3. Create an opening in the occlusal surface of the crown if it is a posterior tooth, or the lingual surface if an anterior (Figs. 7-3, 7-4, and 7-17). This opening should be over the entrance to the canal selected to receive the post, and should meet the criteria for an endodontic access opening in regard to location.

Step 4. Remove the gutta-percha from the desired canal with Peeso Reamers.* The noncutting tip on the Peeso Reamer makes canal perforation an unlikely possibility while the gutta-percha is being removed.[13] Leave a minimum of 3 to 4 mm of root canal filling material for proper apical seal. If the tooth was originally filled with a silver point, remove it if possible, and replace it with gutta-percha.

The post preparation can be completed during the same appointment as the root canal filling without risking damage to the apical seal.[14,15] Remove all gutta-percha from the lateral walls of the canal, and make a radiograph to determine the amount of filling material left in the apical portion of the canal, and to verify the absence of material on the walls. Enlarge the canal using the graduated Peeso Reamers until the proper size of Parapost drill* can be used to hone the canal to fit the selected post.

*Union Broach Co., Long Island City, New York.

*Whaledent International, New York, N.Y.

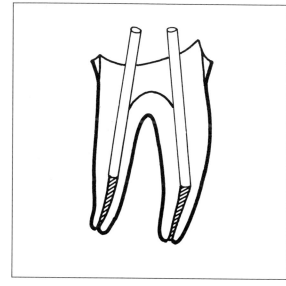

Fig. 7-18 Cross-section of mandibular molar with paraposts in place after preparation of canals.

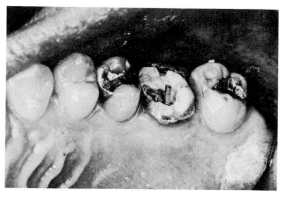

Fig. 7-19 Maxillary molar with parapost cemented in the palatal canal. Post is within walls of initial crown preparation and does not interfere with complete seating of the crown.

Peeso reamer	Parapost drill	Parapost
1	—	—
2	4	4
3	5	5
4	—	—
5	6	6
6	7	7

Try-in the proper post and verify that it is stable and retentive in the canal. Adjust the post length by cutting or bending until it is within the proper axial contours of the proposed preparation, which is dictated by the inner form of the existing crown (Figs. 7-18 and 7-19).

Step 5. Try-in the crown with the uncemented post in place and verify that the post does not interfere with either seating the crown or injecting the composite through the opening in the occlusal or lingual surface. Adjust the post length at its coronal end as necessary.

Step 6. Remove the crown and post, and cement the post. Be certain that cement covers the walls of the full length of the canal by first placing cement in the canal with a periodontal probe, endodontic file, lentulo file, or other simi-

lar instrument. Placing cement on the post prior to seating it may help in wetting the surface irregularities of the post, thereby attaining better retention, but it should not be the only means of introducing cement into the canal. Once it is set, any cement which extruded from the canal into the coronal portion of the tooth should be removed to maximize the strength and retention of the composite buildup.

Step 7. Lightly lubricate the inside of the crown with petroleum jelly or tin-foil substitute. Failure to do this may result in being unable to remove the crown once the composite buildup material has set.

Step 8. Replace the crown on the tooth and stabilize it with either softened compound or acrylic resin. Softened compound can be adapted to the facial and lingual surfaces of the loose crown and the adjacent teeth. This is best done by the assistant so that the dentist can verify with the explorer that the casting is seated perfectly. The importance of this step cannot be overemphasized. It simply is not reliable to attempt to hold the crown in position with the fingers while injecting the buildup material (Fig. 7-20).

Acrylic resin can be used instead of compound to temporarily connect the crown to the adjacent tooth. Place the powder and liquid in separate dappen dishes, and lightly place a small brush in the powder to form a small bead of wet resin. Place this wet resin bead on the marginal ridge of the retainer and the marginal ridge of the adjacent tooth, allowing the material to flow into the interproximal contact area. While the resin is setting, an assistant should hold the crown in proper position manually or with a dental instrument so that the dentist can use an explorer to verify that the casting is perfectly seated. Repeat this procedure on the other marginal ridge (Figs. 7-7 and 7-8).

Step 9. Verify that the seating is complete and the crown is stable. If there is any question, break away the compound stabilizing matrices or acrylic resin and repeat the previous step 8.

Step 10. Mix equal parts base and activator of any conventional (not light-cured) composite material. Inject it through the opening in the crown, being careful that the syringe tip does not totally occlude the opening. If it does the following three problems may ensue:

1. There will be air entrapment, making it difficult for the buildup material to completely fill the inside of the crown.
2. The operator will not be able to tell when the crown is completely filled.
3. Pressure inside the crown may force the crown off the margins, allowing a film of composite between the crown and the finish line of the preparation. This would necessitate removing the entire buildup and repeating the previous steps, since any buildup material left between the margin of the crown and finish line of the tooth will directly cause incomplete seating of the crown.

Eliminate these problems by making sure that the opening is oval, to prevent the round syringe tip from occluding it. Allow buildup material to set completely. Use a coloring agent in the composite, such as black or deep purple, to facilitate the examination of the final buildup, after removing the crown to be absolutely sure that none of the buildup material has extruded

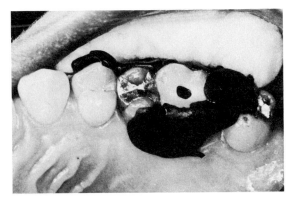

Fig. 7-20 Stabilization with compound of maxillary molar crown in place with margins closed.

between the crown and the tooth at the finish line. Add a coloring agent by rubbing a pencil of the desired color on a mixing pad before mixing the composite. When the composite is mixed over the colored area, the color will be incorporated into the mix. Precolored buildup material is also available from many manufacturers of composite materials.

Step 11. Remove the crown and inspect the buildup for defects such as voids or buildup material on a margin (Figs. 7-21 and 7-22). Small voids may be ignored or filled with composite if desired, but if any material extruded between the crown and the finish line of the preparation, the entire buildup must be removed, saving the post, and steps 7 to 10 repeated. Simply removing the material from the offending area would cause an open margin, since the remaining new buildup will prevent the crown from seating any further. It will often be necessary to drill out the buildup material that set in the access hole before removing the crown. If difficulty is encountered in removing the crown, use a Richwill remover according to directions in chapter 2.

Step 12. Place the crown onto the new buildup and verify the marginal fit as one would at the try-in of any new restoration. The identical criteria must be satisfied as for any other crown.

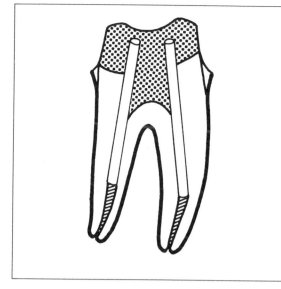

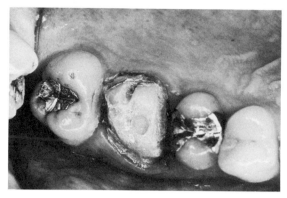

Fig. 7-22 Composite buildup on maxillary molar retained with parapost.

Fig. 7-21 Cross-section of mandibular molar with buildup retained by two paraposts.

Step 13. Remove the crown and clean off any debris, such as the separating medium, with an appropriate solvent. Cement the crown as with any other restoration. The crown will probably be easier to seat completely because it is vented. Special treatment of the opening on a porcelain occlusal surface will be discussed in the next step.

Step 14. Close the access opening in the occlusal surface in one of the following ways:

1. If the crown is gold or porcelain-fused-to-metal with the access through the metal portion, make a Class I preparation by removing all cement to the level of the buildup material. Place either an amalgam or inlay restoration to fill the defect (Figs. 7-23 and 7-24). Restorations involving endodontically treated teeth are discussed in full in chapter 5.

2. If the crown is porcelain-fused-to-metal with access through the porcelain, fill the defect with composite for esthetic purposes. The porcelain part of the preparation should be slightly flared as for the inlay preparation. It is not advisable, nor necessary, to undercut this part of the preparation as for an amalgam or foil, since this would weaken the remaining porcelain. A slight undercut between the metal and buildup material will give some mechanical retention. The key to this procedure is a silane bonding material that will enable the composite to join with the remaining porcelain to make a tight, strong seal. A light-cured composite is recommended for the filling material because of its superior properties and ease of use. Chapters 3 and 5 detail this technique for closing access openings in crowns.

3. Baking porcelain across the defect in the porcelain oven can occasionally be done to close the defect in this area of porcelain-fused-to-metal crowns. This technique has limited usage because of several potential problems. For specific detail regarding this method, as well as its hazards, please refer to page 135.

Method: When the crown has not lost retention

Step 1. Remove all material from the access opening down to the floor of the chamber, such as temporary filling material or gutta-percha. It is important to remove this without weakening the remaining tooth structure.

Step 2. Select which canal or canals should be used for the preformed post. As a first choice,

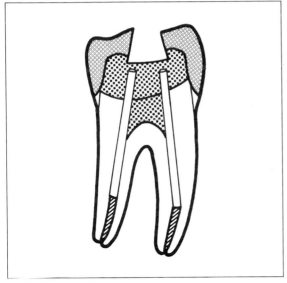

Fig. 7-23 Cross-section of mandibular molar crown over composite buildup with preparation in crown for direct filling material. Walls are slightly undercut.

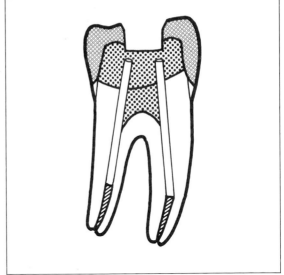

Fig. 7-24 Cross-section of mandibular molar crown over composite buildup with preparation in crown for cast gold inlay. Walls are slightly flared with slight bevel at finish line.

the largest and straightest canal should be used. Generally, this will be the palatal canal in maxillary molars or the distal canal in mandibular molars. In other multirooted teeth, the canal with the most direct access will be the best one to use.

Step 3. Remove the gutta-percha from the desired canal with Peeso Reamers. The noncutting tip on the Peeso Reamer makes canal perforation an unlikely possibility while the gutta-percha is being removed.[13] A minimum of 3 to 4 mm of root canal filling material must be left for proper apical seal. If the tooth was originally filled with silver point, remove it if possible, and replace with gutta-percha. It is very unlikely that this will be possible because of poorer visibility and access to the silver point.

Determine the status of the material used for the initial root canal filling before proceeding. Attempt this technique only rarely in the case of a silver point root canal filling. If it is necessary to redo the root canal filling with gutta-percha, the post preparation can be accomplished at the same appointment as the root canal filling without fear of damage to the apical seal.[14,15] Remove all gutta-percha from the lateral walls of the canal.

Take a radiograph to determine the amount of filling material left in the apical portion of the canal, and verify the absence of material on the walls. Enlarge the canal using the graduated Peeso Reamers until the proper size of Parapost drill can be used to hone the canal to fit the selected post (see chart on page 140). Try in the proper post and verify that it is stable and retentive in the canal. Adjust the post length by cutting or bending until it is within the proper axial contours of the existing crown.

Step 4. Cement the post, being certain that there is cement along the full length of the canal walls by first placing cement in the canal with a periodontal probe, endodontic file, lentulo file, or similar instrument. Placing cement on the post prior to seating it may help in wetting the surface irregularities of the post, thereby attaining slightly better retention. It should not, however, be the only means of introducing cement into the canal. Once set, remove any cement that can be easily reached that has extruded from the canal into the coronal portion of the tooth to maximize the strength and retention of the composite buildup. However, because of limited access and visibility, it is better to leave a small amount of cement in the chamber, rather than risk weakening the post retention by attempting to remove all cement with a handpiece and bur.

Step 5. Mix equal parts base and activator of any conventional (not light-cured) crown buildup composite material. Inject through the opening in the crown, being careful that the syringe tip does not totally occlude the opening. If it does, two problems will possibly ensue: *(1)* Air can be entrapped making it difficult for the buildup material to completely fill the inside of the crown; and *(2)* The operator may be unable to tell when the crown is completely filled.

Step 6. In this case, a coloring agent is not recommended, since this composite will actually be the final restoration in some cases for the access opening. Adjust the occlusion and polish the restoration. If either a silver amalgam or gold inlay is desired, refer to chapter 5 for the recommended technique (Figs. 7-23 and 7-24).

Cast post and core

There are two methods for using cast posts and cores to reinforce previously fabricated castings. The first method can be used when the casting has lost retention and is out of the mouth.

This technique will usually be the treatment of choice in anterior teeth and in premolars when a significant amount of coronal tooth structure has been lost. Anterior teeth, owing either to their funnel-shaped canal orifices or the endodontic procedure itself, often present with canals not suited to preformed posts. Neither a preformed post or a cast post will strengthen the root of the tooth; they are only a means of attaining retention for a crown.

Anterior teeth should receive the best type of post for distributing stress and simultaneously providing adequate retention for the restoration. Studies have shown that this is best achieved using posts of adequate length and minimal diameter.[16] Often, when the original crown was made without a post, a fractured tooth results.

The second is a preventive method to use when successful endodontic therapy is completed through an existing cast restoration with a crown that has not lost retention. It is a modification of a technique advocated by Stackhouse,[17] in which the cast post serves three purposes:

1. Acts to evenly distribute stress.
2. Increases the retention of the previously cemented casting.
3. Becomes the final restoration of the access.

Both methods for the cast post and core require that the existing occlusal relationships, margins, contours, interproximal contacts, and esthetics are acceptable both to the patient and the dentist. Fabricate a new crown if there are any defects.

Method: When the crown can be removed

Step 1. Clean the inside of the crown of any remaining cement, bases, or tooth structure. Remove caries or unsupported tooth structure. Try the crown on the tooth and verify that all margins are present and that the crown is stable, though not necessarily retentive. This step is very important, because margins that are not acceptable beyond question at this point indicate the need for a new crown.

Step 2. Create an opening in the lingual surface of the crown if it is an anterior, or the occlusal if a posterior, which will be over the opening of the canal (Fig. 7-25). Place the crown back on the tooth and verify that the opening is in line with the canal. The opening will then usually meet the criteria for an endodontic access. Put the crown aside.

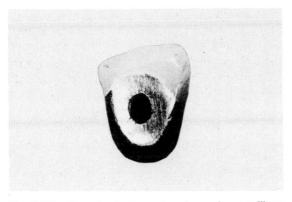

Fig. 7-25 Opening in lingual surface of a maxillary anterior crown that has lost retention because of fracture of the preparation coronal to the finish lines.

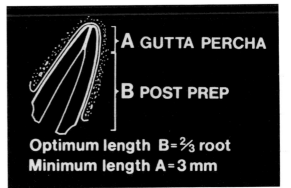

A GUTTA PERCHA

B POST PREP

Optimum length B=⅔ root
Minimum length A=3 mm

Fig. 7-26 Diagrammatic representation of optimum length of post space and minimum length of remaining gutta-percha.

Step 3. Remove the gutta-percha with a Peeso Reamer so that at least 3 to 4 mm of gutta-percha remains in the apical portion of the canal for a good seal (Fig. 7-26). Prepare the canal so that the preparation will have a diameter only large enough for handling materials. Observe requirements for proper stress distribution resulting from adequate length and minimal diameter. If the previous endodontic filling was a silver point, remove it if possible and replace it with a gutta-percha filling. If the old silver point cannot be removed, then the tooth may not be restorable.

Step 4. Fit a plastic toothpick snugly to the canal but not binding. Place several notches in the toothpick for retention of the acrylic. Lightly lubricate the inside of the canal with petroleum jelly, tin-foil substitute, or die lubricant.

Step 5. Make the post portion of the post and core pattern by mixing a self-curing acrylic resin, such as Duralay, and inject it into the canal with a composite syringe, until full. Immediately place the previously adapted toothpick into the canal using one smooth motion. When the acrylic sets to a doughy stage, pump the toothpick and acrylic up and down in the canal two or three times so that it will be easily removed when set. After it has set, verify the stability of this portion in the canal, and be sure

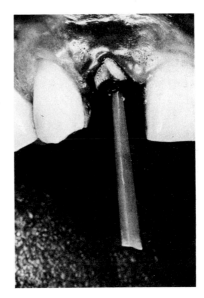

Fig. 7-27 Post portion of acrylic resin pattern, with coronal portion yet to be added.

that it does not move laterally. If such movement occurs, repeat this step (Fig. 7-27).

Step 6. Lightly lubricate the inside of the crown with petroleum jelly, die lubricant or tin-foil substitute. This step is necessary to ensure that the crown and acrylic pattern can later be separated. Trim the coronal portion of the toothpick

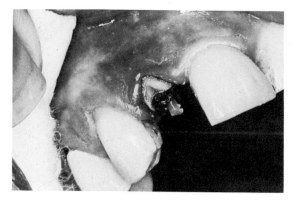

Fig. 7-28 Acrylic resin pattern ready for crown. Neither toothpick nor acrylic resin prevent seating of the crown.

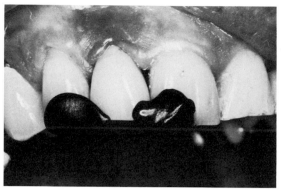

Fig. 7-29 Crown over pattern stabilized with compound.

and acrylic so that the crown can be placed on the tooth over the dowel pattern with all the margins perfectly closed. Ascertain that the post does not interfere in any way with complete seating of the crown (Fig. 7-28). Remove the crown and place notches in the coronal portion of the toothpick.

Step 7. Place the crown on the tooth with the dowel portion of the pattern in place in the root canal preparation, and stabilize it in one of the following ways:

1. Adapt softened compound onto the facial surfaces of the crown and the teeth mesial and distal to it. The importance of this step cannot be overemphasized (Fig. 7-29). It is too risky to attempt to hold the crown in position with the fingers while injecting the buildup material.

2. A second method for stabilizing the crown uses Duralay resin to temporarily connect the adjacent teeth with the crown. Place the powder and liquid in separate dappen dishes. Place a small brush lightly in the powder to form a small bead of wet resin. Place this bead of resin in one facial embrasure, allowing the material to flow into the interproximal contact area (Figs. 7-7 and 7-8). While the resin is setting, hold the crown in proper position with finger or dental instrument. This is best done by the assistant so that the dentist can use an explorer to verify that

the casting is perfectly seated. Repeat this procedure on the other facial embrasure to stabilize the crown while the balance of the pattern is made. It is absolutely essential to reexamine the margins to verify that the crown is securely placed with all the margins perfectly seated. It is risky to attempt to hold the crown in position with the fingers while injecting the buildup material.

Step 8. Mix more acrylic resin and inject it carefully and slowly through the opening on the lingual surface of the crown with the composite syringe until it fills the crown to the opening. Allow the acrylic resin to set completely (Fig. 7-30).

Step 9. Remove both the crown and acrylic resin pattern, and separate them. Remove some of the excess acrylic resin from the lingual opening if necessary. If sufficient lubricant has been used, this is usually not difficult. Carefully inspect the pattern to ensure there are not any voids between the post and core portions (Fig. 7-31).

Step 10. Try the crown and the post and core pattern in the mouth, verifying that the margins are perfectly closed and the crown is stable. If it is impossible to make a needed correction to attain perfect fit of the crown margins, discard the pattern and repeat the procedure. Once this

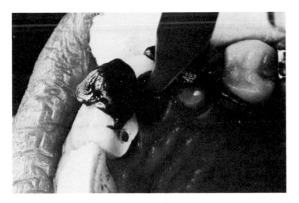

Fig. 7-30 Resin is injected into the crown with composite syringe to complete the pattern.

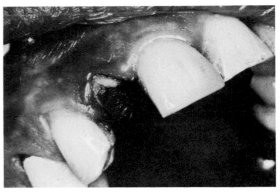

Fig. 7-31 Completed acrylic resin dowel and core pattern.

is accomplished, put the acrylic pattern and the crown aside and temporize the tooth with a polycarbonate crown and a temporary acrylic post.

Step 11. Invest, burnout, and cast the post and core pattern in the usual manner. Since the post should be slightly smaller than the canal to avoid undesirable stresses on seating, use 1 to 2 cc more water than is usually used with the investment. After removing all investment from the casting, clean the casting and try the core in the crown. Use the microscope to determine that the post and crown fit back together properly, and that nothing interferes with complete seating of the two components. Any undetected error will cause an open margin when the crown is later seated in the mouth. Use a mixture of chloroform and gold rouge painted on the core before assembling the two parts to identify any areas of interference. Once this step is completed, the post and crown can be tried in the mouth.

Step 12. Try the dowel in the mouth, assess completeness of seating, and adjust as necessary to gain complete seating (Fig. 7-32). Any incomplete seating at this stage will cause an open margin of the final crown; *complete seating is essential.* When you are satisfied that the

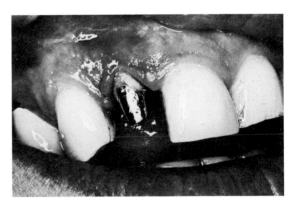

Fig. 7-32 Cast dowel seated in tooth.

post fits perfectly, try-in the crown and verify that the margins are closed and that the interproximal and occlusal contacts are proper. Make any necessary adjustments.

Step 13. Seat the post with a permanent cement and remove all excess cement. Again, verify that the crown still fits and then cement the crown with a permanent cement (Fig. 7-33).

Step 14. Finally, remove the cement which has extruded from the opening on the lingual or occlusal surface with an inverted cone bur. This will cause an undercut preparation. Restore the

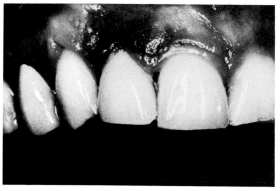

Fig. 7-33 Crown adjusted and cemented on new dowel core.

access opening in the occlusal or lingual surface by one of the following methods:

1. If the crown is gold or porcelain-fused-to-metal with access through the metal portion, make a Class I preparation removing all cement to the level of the buildup material. Either an amalgam or inlay restoration may be used to fill the defect (Figs. 7-23 and 7-24). See chapter 5 on restorations involving endodontically treated teeth for more detail on this procedure.

2. If the crown is porcelain-fused-to-metal with access through the porcelain, the defect can be filled with composite for esthetic purposes. Slightly flare the preparation as for an inlay preparation. It is neither advisable nor necessary to undercut the porcelain part of the crown, since this would weaken the remaining porcelain. However, a slight undercut of the underlying metal will enhance retention. The key to this procedure is the silane bonding material, which will enable the composite to join with the remaining porcelain in a tight, strong seal.

   A light cured composite is a superior filling material, and is easier to use than conventional composites. For greater detail on the use of silane and composite for closing access openings in crowns, please refer to chapters 3 and 5 on correction of facings and endodontic procedures under existing restorations.

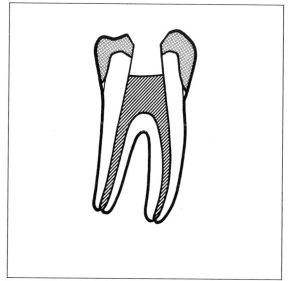

Fig. 7-34 Crown on endodontically treated tooth with bevelled margins around access opening.

3. Occasionally, defects in the porcelain area of porcelain-fused-to-metal crowns can also be closed by baking porcelain across them. This, unlike the other methods, requires a laboratory procedure as well as a subsequent office visit. In many cases, this will not be the method of choice because of several potential problems. For specific detail regarding this method, as well as its hazards, refer to page 135.

Method: Crown cannot or has not been removed

Step 1. Enlarge the occlusal or lingual opening in the crown to provide good visibility and access. Place a wide bevel on the occlusal surface for finishing and for preventing apical displacement of the post and the attendant risk of root stress (Fig. 7-34).

Step 2. Remove any debris and gutta-percha from the pulp chamber with a hot instrument and/or a no. 4 or no. 6 round bur. Particular care should be exercised not to create undercuts or weaken any remaining tooth structure.

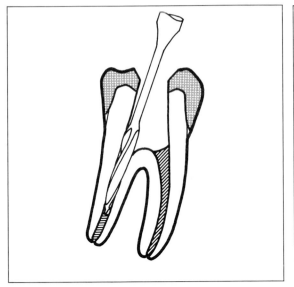

Fig. 7-35 Peeso reamer used to remove gutta-percha and shape canal walls.

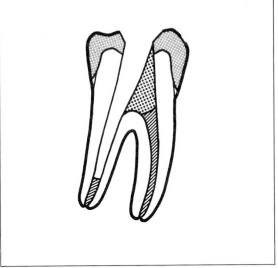

Fig. 7-36 Undercuts in pulp chamber blocked out with composite material.

Step 3. Select the canal that will receive the post. In maxillary molars, the palatal root is usually the best while in mandibular molars, the distal root is usually best. In maxillary first premolars, either root is usually adequate.

Step 4. Remove the gutta-percha and enlarge the canal if the endodontist has not done this already. This is most easily and safely done with a Peeso Reamer in a slow-speed handpiece. Prepare the canal so that at least 3 to 4 mm of gutta-percha remains in the canal at the apical end for a good seal (Fig. 7-35). The diameter of the canal should only be large enough for the materials to be properly handled, recognizing the requirement for proper stress distribution resulting from adequate length and minimal diameter. Carefully ascertain that the walls of the canal are not perforated. If there is any uncertainty about the location or direction of the canal, either take additional radiographs or enlarge the access opening to be certain of proper instrumentation.

Step 5. Block out all undercuts and irregularities in the pulp chamber. If the chamber is not large

or the undercuts are minimal, simply place zinc phosphate cement or composite resin inside the pulp chamber, and smooth it with a smooth hand instrument such as a Gregg* no. 4/5 (Fig. 7-36). However, if the chamber is large with several irregular or undercut areas, an alternate procedure is necessary. First, select a wire such as a paperclip or an orthodontic wire and ensure that it can be inserted in the canal to the full length. For the wire to properly fit into the apical portion of the canal, it may need to be beveled at the end. Lubricate and insert the wire into the canal to the apical end. Prepare a thin mix of zinc phosphate cement and fill the upper end of the canal and most of the pulp chamber. As the cement sets, move the wire with a rotating motion to prepare a straight, smooth, divergent channel from the apical end of the canal to the opening of the crown. Remove the wire after the cement sets.

Step 6. Use a Peeso Reamer to ream and smooth the length of the channel just formed,

*Columbus Dental, St. Louis, Mo.

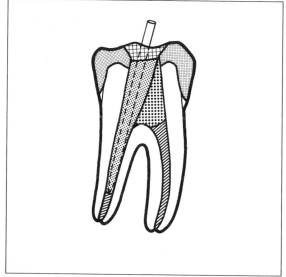

Fig. 7-37 Dowel core pattern of self-curing resin and inlay wax in occlusal portion around plastic toothpick.

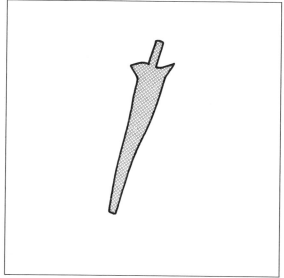

Fig. 7-38 Cast dowel core with part of sprue attached to use as a handle.

and remove any cement or filling material from the original access with a bur or stone. Select and taper a plastic toothpick to fit in the channel to the apical end. Extend the toothpick out of the occlusal or lingual opening several millimeters to easily handle the material. Place retentive notches in the toothpick and lubricate the length of the preparation with petroleum jelly, die lube, or tin-foil substitute.

Step 7. Fabricate the post pattern by mixing self-curing acrylic resin and injecting it into the prepared channel with a composite syringe until it is completely filled. Immediately insert the previously selected toothpick into the resin to the apical end of the channel with one smooth motion. When the acrylic sets to a doughy stage, pump the toothpick and acrylic up and down in the channel two or three times to ensure that it can be easily removed when set. After it has set, verify that the pattern in the canal is stable, with no lateral movement, and no defects or voids. If there is lateral movement, repeat this step after selecting a new toothpick and relubricating the channel.

Step 8. When the internal section of the pattern has been satisfactorily fabricated, the occlusal or lingual portion of the post must be made of inlay wax. Remove excess resin but retain the toothpick to provide a handle with which to remove the pattern. Add soft inlay wax to the occlusal portion of the pattern and carve this flush with existing contours (Fig. 7-37). Occlusion can only be approximated because the toothpick is present. Final occlusion will need to be adjusted in the casting after cementation.

Step 9. Invest, burnout, and cast in the usual manner, but with a Class I gold alloy which will allow for a greater degree of marginal adaptation in the finished casting. As with all cast posts, use 1 or 2 cc more water to make the post small enough to preclude stress in the root. After casting, clean the post and check carefully for defects in the casting with a microscope. Leaving the sprue attached for the try-in can be very helpful as a handle (Fig. 7-38).

Step 10. Using a hemostat to hold the casting by the sprue, try it in the mouth to verify complete

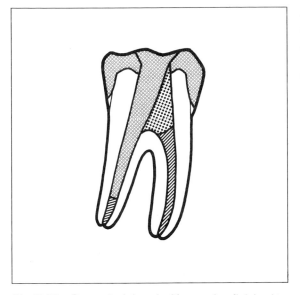

Fig. 7-39 Cemented dowel with margins finished to original casting.

Step 11. After the post is adapted to the canal, cut partly through the sprue until a small amount of gold attaches the post to the sprue. Mix zinc phosphate cement and apply it to all the walls of the prepared channel with a periodontal probe, a root canal explorer, or a lentulo spiral. While holding the sprue, coat the post with cement and seat it into the channel. Use a hemostat to remove the sprue with a twisting motion, and have the patient bite on a wooden stick while the cement sets. After the cement has set, adjust the occlusion, add any necessary occlusal anatomy, and polish with rubber points (Fig. 7-39).

Using a one-piece cast inlay and post helps to prevent fracturing of teeth that have had endodontic therapy after a crown or bridge was cemented. It also provides additional retention of the crown or bridge because of the bevel at the occlusal surface and the second line of draw provided by the post. This is important in terms of post-cementation endodontics on one abutment of a bridge. Without this reinforcement, one retainer could become loose and cause rapid deterioration of the abutment. Since the tooth is not vital, the deterioration may render it unrestorable without ever producing any symptoms.

seating, well-adapted margins, and snugness of fit. Use chloroform and rouge painted on the casting to find any areas of interference when the casting is tried in the canal. Reduce areas where rouge is worn through until seating is complete with all margins closed.

References

1. Asawa, G.N. Cast dowel core fabrication on a preexisting crown. Dent. Surg. 48:36–37, 1972.
2. Federick, D.R. An application of the dowel and composite resin core technique. J. Prosthet. Dent. 32:420–424, 1974.
3. Goldstein, R.E. Esthetics in Dentistry. Philadelphia: J.B. Lippincott Co., 1976, pp. 292–295.
4. Ogesen, R.B. Reusing a crown from a fractured tooth. Dent. Dig. 536–539, 1967.
5. Portera, J.J., and Thomson, J.A. Reuse of existing crown after tooth fracture at the gingival margin. J. Prosthet. Dent. 50:195–197, 1983.
6. Priest, G., and Goerig, A. Post and core fabrication beneath an existing crown. J. Prosthet. Dent. 42:645–648, 1979.
7. Richardson, J.T., and Padgett, J.G. Repair technique for a fractured, crowned anterior tooth. J. Prosthet. Dent. 31:409–410, 1974.
8. Richardson, J.T., and Sox, J.T. Repair technique for a fractured crowned tooth. J. Prosthet. Dent. 37:547–549, 1977.
9. Rothenberg, M.S. The crown that failed and how to save it. Dent. Surg. 1970.
10. Shirdel, K., et al. Construction of a post and core to fit a completed restoration. J. Prosthet. Dent. 38.229–231, 1977.
11. Dewhirst, R.B., et al. Dowel-core fabrication. J. S. Cal. Dent. Assoc. 37(10):444–449, 1969.
12. Brady, W.F. Restoration of a tooth to accommodate a preexisting cast crown. J. Prosthet. Dent. 48:268–270, 1982.
13. Fisher, D.W., et al. An evaluation of methods for preparing teeth to receive retentive posts. J. Dent. Res. 61:237, 1982.
14. Bourgeois, R.S., and Lemon, R.R. Dowel space preparation and apical leakage. J. Endo. 7:66–69, 1981.
15. Kwan, E.H., and Harrington, G.W. The effect of immediate post preparation on apical seal. J. Endo. 7:325–329, 1981.

16. Caputo, A.A., and Standlee, J.P. Pins and posts—Why, when, and how. D. Clin. N. Am. 20:299, 1976.
17. Stackhouse, J.A. Reinforcement of nonvital crowned teeth. J. Am. Dent. Assoc. 104:859–861, 1982.

Additional reading

Beheshti, N. Fabricating a post and core to fit an existing crown. J. Prosthet. Dent. 42:236–239, 1979.

Cooney, J.P. Coronal buildup procedures. Fixed Prosthodontic Syllabus (unpublished). Los Angeles: University of California School of Dentistry, 1978.

Federick, D.R. An application of the dowel and composite resin core technique. J. Prosthet. Dent. 32:420–424, 1974.

Frank, A.L. Protective coronal coverage of the pulpless tooth. J. Am. Dent. Assoc. 59:895–900, 1959.

Henry, P.J., and Bower, R.C. Secondary intention post and core. Aust. Dent. J. 22:128–131, 1977.

Ingle, J. Endodontics. Philadelphia: Lea & Febiger, 1965, pp. 612–631.

Lovdahl, P.E., and Dumont, T.D. A dowel core technique for multirooted teeth. J. Prosthet. Dent. 27:44–47, 1972.

Perel, M.L., and Muroff, F.I. Clinical criteria for posts and cores, J. Prosthet. Dent. 28:405–411, 1972.

Rosen, H. Operative procedures on mutilated endodontically treated teeth. J. Prosthet. Dent. 11:973–986, 1961.

Samani, S.I.A., and Harris, W.T. A procedure for repairing fractured post-core restorations. J. Prosthet. Dent. 39:627–631, 1978.

Shillingburg, H.T., and Kessler, J.C. Restoration of the Endodontically Treated Tooth. Chicago: Quintessence Publ. Co., 1982.

Shillingburg, H.T., et al. Restoration of endodontically treated posterior teeth. J. Prosthet. Dent. 24:401–409, 1970.

Steele, G.D. Reinforced composite resin foundations for endodontically treated teeth. J. Prosthet. Dent. 30:816–819, 1973.

Waliszewski, K.J., and Sabala, C.L. Combined endodontic and restorative treatment considerations. J. Prosthet. Dent. 40:152–156, 1978.

Chapter 8

Modifications to Removable Appliances

Many people wear partial dentures with which they are quite satisfied. One problem in dealing with defects in existing dentures is that the same level of satisfaction may be difficult to attain again, at least in the mind of a patient who has become accustomed to the idiosyncracies of his or her restoration and prefers not to disturb the status quo. But the difference in the cost of replacing the restoration in its entirety versus correcting the problem by modifying the existing restoration will make modification the treatment of choice for some patients.

The techniques presented in this chapter for restoring the removable appliances themselves are those the authors have found to result in restorations of the same high quality and function as the originals, if not better.

It is axiomatic that more questionable procedures are attempted when patients present with defects in removable appliances than when problems are found with cemented restorations. This can be justified in many ways, depending on a clinician's bias regarding the permanence of partial dentures and their potential effects on the remaining oral structures. *A properly designed, well-constructed, and diligently maintained removable partial denture is a permanent restoration and should not be considered as a step toward full dentures.*[1] Unfortunately, too many partial dentures have been designed and constructed to be temporary. Modifications to these appliances over the years tend to be makeshift.

Accordingly, some of the procedures described in this chapter are of a slightly different nature than the others dealt with in this book. For example, relining a distal-extension partial denture might not be done to remedy a defect in the denture itself, but to accommodate a change in the bone contour.

Refer to chapter 4 for a discussion of the principles of partial denture design and consider these when deciding whether to modify or remake a restoration. It is important to weigh design principles on two fronts:

1. If a denture is not designed so that it is properly serviceable, the need for a corrective procedure can be taken as an opportunity to promote the potential benefits of constructing an entirely new denture.

2. A modification could result in a partial denture that no longer satisfies the requirements for a successful restoration. For example: assume that an abutment tooth for a distal extension partial denture needs to be extracted. A clasp that would attach to the next tooth in the arch could be added to the partial denture. However, this second abutment tooth might not satisfy the same mechanical or biological requirements as the extracted tooth did years before when the decision was made to use it as the abutment. This new abutment tooth may be periodontally involved or may not have proper contour to provide positive occlusal rest. In this case, it would not suffice simply to modify the partial by adding a new clasp.

The partial denture, as with any other restoration to be corrected, must be perfect or correctable in all other respects. The difference, however, between partial dentures and fixed restorations in this regard is that it can be justifiable to correct more than one defect in the partial denture. For example, when replacing a clasp which has broken off of an old partial denture, it is often observed that the restoration needs a reline on one or more saddle areas. Neither of these defects taken alone would normally require remaking the partial denture. It follows then that both corrections could be made on the same partial denture, since the need for a reline has no effect on the clasp replacement and, conversely, the reline can be done just as well after the clasp is corrected as it could be if the clasp were in perfect condition to begin with.

As will be the case with many corrections to existing partial dentures, the primary work will be accomplished in the laboratory, rather than at chairside, as with a facing replacement on a fixed restoration. However, the role played by the dentist is extremely important. The dentist must make impressions that generate casts with which the technician will be able to perform the necessary procedures, evaluate the suitability of the partial presented for correcting, and make adjustments to the denture prior to making impressions. Otherwise, even though the cast may be generally acceptable to the laboratory, the correction may be impossible due to a small oversight. These specific problems will be pointed out later as procedures are presented.

Addition of metal occlusal surfaces

It may be advisable to convert the standard acrylic denture teeth to cast metal occlusal surfaces for either of the following reasons:

1. To attain better control of the occlusion by actually waxing the cusps against a mounted cast of the opposing occlusal surfaces.

2. To decrease or eliminate the wear caused by bruxism, which could be leading to a decrease in vertical dimension or loss of a stable centric occlusal (CO) position.

Adding metal occlusal surfaces is not often called for, but when it is it can make the difference between a partial denture that will frequently need replacement or modification, and one that will have longevity.

Some methods advocated in dental literature involve making castings with facings of tooth-colored resin retained by new acrylic locking around bars in the castings,[2] while others require pin-retained castings.[3]

The method described below deals with a mandibular partial denture. Before proceeding, the patient should wear a new partial long enough for any needed adjustments to arise, though the occlusion itself need only be adequate enough not to be causing tissue irritation, since it will be replaced in the procedure.

Method

Step 1

Verify that the partial denture perfectly fits the abutment teeth, has adequate retention, and does not need a reline. If any of these defects are present, they must be taken care of before proceeding. Here only the stability of both the denture base and the metal framework is important, not the occlusion. In this procedure, it is important that the acrylic distal extension saddle areas are in good tissue contact. The reason for this is that an occlusal registration will be made using the partial denture.

Step 2

Remove the acrylic from the occlusal surfaces of the denture teeth such that when the restoration is placed in the mouth, there will be occlusal clearance in centric position of at least 2 mm. This reduction should be done on a flat plane rather than by reproducing the inclines, as

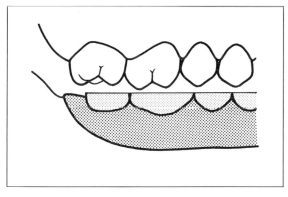

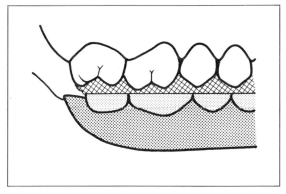

Fig. 8-1   The occlusal surfaces of the acrylic teeth have been removed from the partial denture, leaving adequate clearance for waxing up new occlusal surfaces and a flat plane.

Fig. 8-2   An interocclusal record at occlusal vertical dimension registering the relationship between the newly developed plane on the partial denture and the opposing teeth.

would be done on a preparation on a natural tooth (Fig. 8-1). In this manner, the pinholes which will retain the occlusal casting will all be drilled into a flat plane, making this procedure easier.

Step 3

Make an occlusal registration in centric position with a zinc oxide and eugenol bite registration paste* or other stable compound. Place the material on the prepared surfaces of the denture teeth and have the patient close the remaining teeth into CO. If there are no other teeth in contact, as in bilateral distal extension cases, then use the same method of positioning the mandible for this registration that was used when the denture was initially made (Fig. 8-2). The advantage of creating the occlusal clearance prior to making the occlusal registration is that the registration can be made while the mandible is at correct occlusal vertical position. This eliminates the error caused when an open-bite record is made and the maxillary cast is not mounted on the true terminal hinge axis.

Step 4

Make protrusive records for correctly setting the

*Kerr/Sybron Manufacturing Co., Romulus, Mich.

semiadjustable or fully adjustable articulator. This step is important in establishing the angles of the eminentia on the articulator. The lower side of the protrusive registration will be imprinted with the form of the bite registration paste that was placed on the dentures in step 3. Though this part of the procedure is unusual, the protrusive record cannot be made using the occlusal anatomy of the partial denture teeth because that anatomy will have been removed by the time the case must be mounted and the articulator adjusted. The bite registration paste or compound is strong enough to endure this procedure without distortion, leaving the centric record intact.

Step 5

Make a full-arch impression over the occlusal registration using irreversible hydrocolloid, with the partial denture in place (Fig. 8-3). Remove the impression with the partial denture in place if possible. If the partial denture remains in the mouth, place it into the impression, and trim away areas, such as those around clasps, that might interfere with proper seating into the impression.

Step 6

Pour this impression with a densite stone, taking

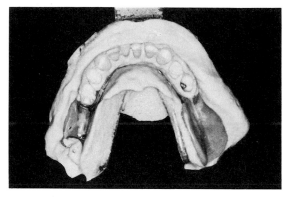

Fig. 8-3 Irreversible hydrocolloid overimpression with partial denture in place.

into account the following modification of the normal impression-pouring technique:

1. Block out any undercuts in the acrylic saddle areas with a standard blockout wax.
2. Reinforce any abutment teeth that may be broken off when the partial denture is removed from the stone cast. This can be done by placing a brass dowel pin or a stiff wire into the impression of the tooth prior to pouring the stone cast.
3. Lightly lubricate the tissue surface of the acrylic saddles with a tin-foil substitute* so the stone will not adhere.

Make an impression for an opposing cast and pour in dental stone.

Step 7

Mount the maxillary cast using a face-bow and mount the mandibular cast using the occlusal registration. The occlusal registration is actually on the partial denture that in turn is attached to the mandibular cast. Set the articulator to the protrusive records, and remove the bite registration paste from the partial denture teeth.

Step 8

Retention is by pins in the casting. Place an adequate number of pinholes parallel to each

other in the acrylic denture teeth. The holes must all be parallel, and this can usually be done by eye. If a paralleling device is needed, use the Ney,* which holds a handpiece on the surveyor. While many different pin systems are available, the authors prefer the VIP (Fig. 8-4). It is composed of a twist drill, an impression pin, a pin for temporaries (not applicable here), and an iridio-platinum pin that will become part of the casting. Generally, two or three pins in each tooth are sufficient, but the number will vary with the anticipated lateral stress from occlusion as well as with the size of the teeth. The pinholes should be 2 mm deep.

This procedure does not involve the VIP system in its entirety. Normally, the impression pins are used in the pinholes of a natural tooth, and the iridio-platinum pins are placed in the holes of the stone cast, which result from pouring stone around the impression pins.

In this method, however, use the holes in the acrylic teeth, which were actually drilled with the twist drill, to position the iridio-platinum pins. Since the size of the parts of this system gradually decreases, the iridio-platinum pins will not be as stable during waxing as they usually would be. This results from the fact that normally the iridio-platinum pins are inserted into holes in a stone cast generated by the impression pins, which are smaller than the holes in these plastic teeth. The size variance for the VIP system is as follows:

Drill, 0.024 mm
Impression pin, 0.017 mm
Iridio-platinum pin, 0.007 mm

Solve this problem by ensuring that all the pins are placed as far as possible in the same direction—in effect, prestressed. Lubricate the surfaces of the acrylic denture teeth that will be contacted by the waxup.

Step 9

Place the iridio-platinum pins in the holes drilled into the acrylic teeth (Fig. 8-5). Close the articulator into CO and verify that none of the pins are

*Alcote, L. D. Caulk Co., Milford, Del.

*J. M. Ney Co., Bloomfield, Conn.

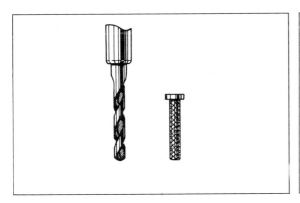

Fig. 8-4 Drill and iridio-platinum pin from Pindex system.

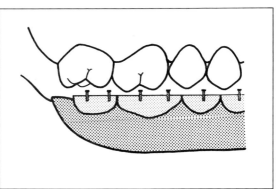

Fig. 8-5 High-fusing metal pins in holes drilled into plastic partial denture teeth. Note there is clearance between all pins and the opposing occlusal surface.

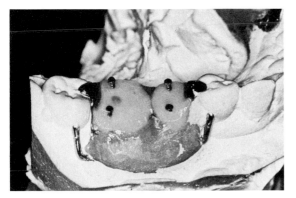

Fig. 8-6a Four pins in place ready for waxing.

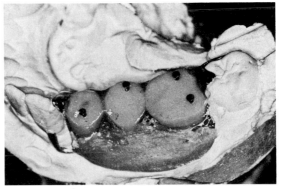

Fig. 8-6b Four pins would also usually be adequate in this three-unit occlusal surface.

long enough to interfere with closure. It is best to reduce the length of the pins below the proposed occlusal surface of the final casting. While a pin visible on the surface after the casting does not present problems, it can create a potential area of roughness that might be hard to finish (Figs. 8-6a and b).

Step 10

Wax the new occlusal surfaces and verify that the occlusion is free of lateral interferences as with any waxup involving the occlusion. This precaution is particularly significant in distal-extension partial denture cases, since a primary goal is always to maintain the health of the bone (Fig. 8-7).

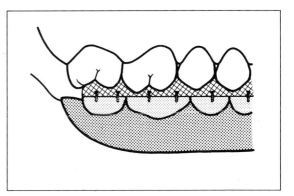

Fig. 8-7 Waxup of new occlusal surfaces for mandibular partial denture.

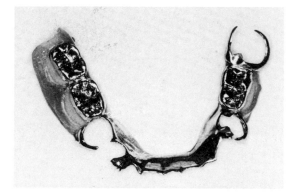

Fig. 8-8 Gold occlusal surfaces on partial denture.

Improvement of retention by modification of axial contour

Occasionally, you may discover upon insertion of a newly constructed partial denture framework that the amount of undercut is insufficient for proper functioning of a retentive clasp (Fig. 8-9). While not a common situation, this can often be easily corrected without remaking the framework. When deciding whether such a simple correction is possible, consider whether the clasp is a circumferential or an I bar type. If it is a circumferential clasp, it may be possible to bend the active tip into an area of greater undercut. This is not possible with the I bar, without risking alteration of its function or the forces it exerts on the abutment tooth.

.Surface material in the area of the undercut itself will be one of the following:

Step 11

Attach multiple sprues in areas of least occlusal contact. Attaching them to either the facial or lingual surfaces of the wax pattern reduces the amount of occlusal adjustment needed later. The various occlusal surfaces are usually waxed and cast in one unit for each saddle area, to ensure the best retention. Cast in a precious, semiprecious, or nonprecious alloy.

1. Natural tooth enamel
2. Gold crown
3. Porcelain facing on a crown
4. Gold inlay
5. Gold foil
6. Silver amalgam
7. Composite resin or other plastic material
8. Acrylic facing on a crown

Only natural tooth enamel and gold crowns are good candidates for the procedure described here. Porcelain facing on a crown, gold inlay, gold foil and silver amalgam are often possibilities, but more care is needed in case selection. Modifying a porcelain facing breaks the glaze, even though it can sometimes be polished with a porcelain polishing system.* The gold inlay or gold foil can develop marginal problems if the clasp functions over the margin after the modification.

Step 12

Check the fit of the casting to the acrylic denture teeth. If all the pins are parallel and the casting is accurate, it should seat completely. If not, careful inspection will likely reveal poor parallelism of the pins. The best course of action in such a case is to drill a new hole in the denture tooth to replace the incorrect one, and to redo the pattern and recast. Do not remove any of the pins—they are all needed, or they should not have been placed.

Determine the function of a clasp under consideration. For example, occasionally a nonretentive facial clasp is designed for a particular tooth, usually in a situation with only one distal extension, and a molar abutment on the other

Step 13

Try the denture in the mouth with the uncemented casting in position on the acrylic teeth. Adjust the occlusion, and polish and cement the casting using either a zinc phosphate cement or a composite luting agent (Fig. 8-8).

*Shofu Dental Corp., Menlo Park, Calif.

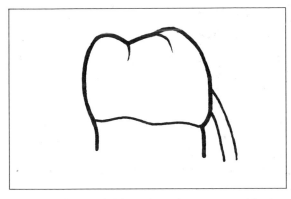

Fig. 8-9 Face of I bar clasp in contact with the surface of the tooth that does not provide adequate retention.

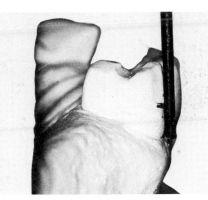

Fig. 8-10 Cast on surveyor using undercut gauge to evaluate original line of draw of the partial denture.

side. Increasing the retention under such conditions could cause problems with the stability of the abutment tooth.

Both gold foil and amalgam are too soft for clasp retention, while neither composite resin nor acrylic is resilient enough to endure the constant abrasion of the clasp as it functions in and out of the undercut.

Most methods presented in dental literature involve changing the contour of the abutment tooth, either by reducing the surface of the tooth or by adding the needed contour with acid etch composites.[4,5,6] The method presented here involves modifying the tooth contour itself without adding any new material.

Method

Step 1

Carefully examine retention of the partial denture in the mouth, focusing on its function in various excursive movements. A restoration will often appear stable in centric position, only to tip or rock out of position during other mandibular movements. Have the patient bite on a cotton roll placed over various points on the partial denture—rests or saddles. If the denture moves when force is applied to an occlusal rest, seriously consider making a new framework. Direct

force applied to an occlusal rest should not cause the framework to tip.

Step 2

Remove the partial denture and make an impression for a full-arch cast. Pour in a dental stone mixed with a plaster slurry to accelerate the set. This cast should be ready for use in 5 minutes.

Step 3

Place the cast on the table of the surveyor and identify the original survey line (Fig. 8-10). This step goes most quickly when the locations of the various undercuts into which the clasps of the partial denture engage are marked on the cast. In the mouth, paint a mixture of gold rouge and chloroform on the facial surface of each tooth upon which a retentive clasp functions. Then place the partial denture in position in the mouth. Each of the clasps will mark through the rouge and chloroform coating and show the most gingival aspect of the travel of the clasp on the surface. This aids primarily in estimating the depth needed for improved retention.

Step 4

Transfer these marks from the mouth to the cast on the surveyor table and adjust the position of the cast accordingly, setting the table so that

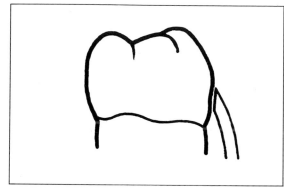

Fig. 8-11 Face of I bar clasp in same position after recontouring of facial surface.

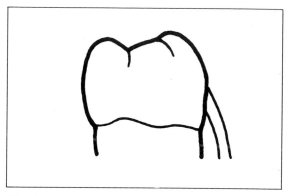

Fig. 8-12 I bar readjusted to function in newly created undercut after alteration of tooth contour.

each mark extends approximately 1 mm gingival to the survey line. This is similar to the relationship between the retentive clasp tip and the survey line in the mouth. At this point it will be relatively easy to judge the degree of undercut attainable on the tooth. A cast helps the clinician to better visualize and plan the modification; miscalculation could make it impossible to attain the necessary undercut.

Step 5

Use the mark as a guide in the mouth to recontour the facial surface such that when the partial denture is in place, the retentive face of the clasp is no longer in contact with the tooth surface. In some cases, this distance may be but a few tenths of a millimeter, while in others it may be more. Recontour such that the degree of undercut in the surface is proper for the clasp to function. Occasionally, this causes a depression in the surface, but more often the change in contour will be barely identifiable visually in the mouth (Fig. 8-11).

Step 6

Remove the partial denture from the mouth, and use standard clasp adjusting technique to bend the retentive portion of the clasp into the undercut (Fig. 8-12). There is a limit to the number of times and the distance a chrome-cobalt clasp

can be bent without it breaking. Try in the partial denture, and carefully examine the contact between the face of the clasp and the tooth surface. Particularly with I bars, adjust this face to attain good contact (Figs. 8-13a and b). Magnification is very helpful during this step.

Step 7

Determine whether the retention has been improved adequately. If not, one of the following actions will be required:

1. Repeat step 5 to create a greater degree of undercut.
2. Further adjust the clasp if necessary.
3. Adjust the angle of the face of the retentive clasp for better contact.

Polish the surface of the tooth or restoration.

Replacement of a broken occlusal rest

A rest will sometimes fracture at the junction with a strut or a proximal plate, depending on the design of the partial denture. The cause can be a casting defect in a case where there is adequate occlusal clearance and the casting is sufficiently thick, or a rest that is too thin due to insufficient clearance.

This procedure requires careful planning because the partial denture framework may have lost the stability required when performing any correction to the metal work. The correction will be successful only if the framework is perfectly stabilized in the mouth while the impression is made over it. The resulting working cast is a composite of the partial denture and the remaining natural dentition in a perfect relationship. A missing occlusal rest can make this difficult or impossible because it is the rests that provide necessary stability. If the necessary stability is not present, do not attempt this correction.

For techniques such as electrowelding of chrome-cobalt partial denture frameworks, be aware of your laboratory's capabilities and limitations. Although dentists tend to work with one laboratory exclusively, special needs may justify, even require, that you seek the services of another laboratory.

Most of these additions or corrections of occlusal rests are done on chrome-cobalt frameworks by electrowelding or electrosoldering techniques. An 0.800 fine solder is used by the laboratory with an electrosoldering device. The resulting joint will be at least 85% as strong as the original casting.[7]

Method

Step 1

Place the partial denture in the mouth and check the fit of all attachments, paying particular attention to whether the denture is stable without the missing rest. The denture may not be stable when placed under its occlusal load, but it must be at least stable enough to maintain perfect position during the impression procedure.

Step 2

With the denture in place, carefully examine the area of failure and bear in mind that the more preparation of the immediate area that can be made by the dentist, the better. For example, if the occlusal rest fractured because the initial preparation was too shallow, and thus the rest

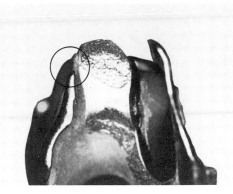

Fig. 8-13a   Face of I bar clasp before adjustment of angle.

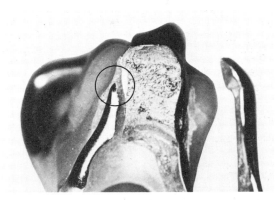

Fig. 8-13b   Face of I bar clasp after adjustment of angle so that clasp can function in newly created undercut.

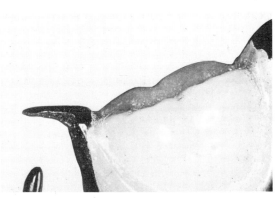

Fig. 8-14   Occlusal rest that was too thin, often due to lack of occlusal clearance.

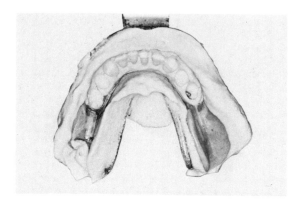

Fig. 8-15a Partial denture in overimpression of irreversible hydrocolloid.

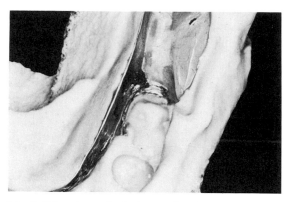

Fig. 8-15b Area of missing occlusal rest. This is the most important part of the impression, in that there must be a perfect impression of the tooth right up to the area of the partial denture where the failure has occurred.

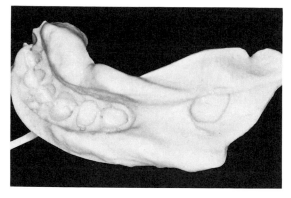

Fig. 8-16 Quadrant impression of the involved tooth needing a new occlusal rest, without the partial denture in place.

too thin (Fig. 8-14), deepen the rest in the abutment tooth if possible before making the impression, so that this relatively common mistake will not be repeated.

Smoothing and recontouring the fractured area of the partial denture is also recommended before sending a case to the laboratory.

Step 3

Make a full-arch irreversible hydrocolloid impression with the partial denture in place, and accurately reproduce the occlusal rest in the abutment tooth. A thinner-than-normal mix of alginate reduces the risk of displacing the partial denture from the pressure of the material while the tray is going into position (Figs. 8-15a and b).

Step 4

Remove this full-arch impression. Usually, the partial denture will come out with the impression and will remain in perfect position, ready for the cast to be poured. However, if it does remain in the mouth, the dentist, rather than the technician, should take the responsibility for placing the partial denture correctly into the impression. Occasionally, it will be necessary to remove small areas of alginate that interfere with clasp areas in order to place the partial in the impression. This is of little concern because this impression requires only that the denture be completely seated when it is poured and that the immediate area of the correction be a perfect reproduction of the conditions in the mouth.

Step 5

Make a second irreversible alginate impression of the area of the correction without the partial denture in place. This impression can be in a simple quadrant tray and will be used to make the wax pattern in some cases (Fig. 8-16).

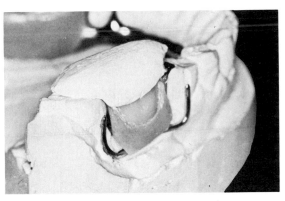

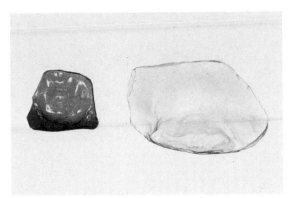

Fig. 8-17 Plaster occlusal index relating the acrylic denture tooth to the adjacent teeth on the cast.

Fig. 8-18 Plaster occlusal index and plastic denture tooth after removal of the tooth from the partial denture.

Step 6

If the laboratory is nearby, send the impressions there for pouring as it is usually best to have the technicians who will ultimately be responsible for waxing and assembling the case also pour the impression. If this arrangement is not possible, the dentist should pour the cast in a densite stone such as Vel Mix.* When pouring the impression, consider the following:

1. Use a standard blockout wax to block out any undercut in the acrylic saddle areas, except for any saddle adjacent to the area where the new occlusal rest will be welded to the partial denture. This acrylic will need to be removed anyway, and when it is replaced it will be important that the cast accurately reproduce the contour of the patient's ridge.
2. Reinforce any abutment teeth that could be broken off when the partial denture is removed from the stone cast. This can be done by simply placing a brass dowel pin (Ney)** or a stiff wire into the impression of the tooth in question before pouring the stone cast.
3. Lightly lubricate the tissue of the acrylic saddle with a tin-foil substitute so the stone will not adhere.

*Kerr/Sybron Manufacturing Co., Romulus, Mich.
**J. M. Ney Co., Bloomfield, Conn.

Step 7

The laboratory technician performs the following procedure, described here in brief so that clinicians might maintain an overview of the entire process:

1. The partial denture is removed from the cast and a refractory cast is made to be used later in the welding operation.
2. If there is acrylic work close to the area to be electrowelded, an occlusal index is made in plaster to relate the denture tooth to the remainder of the teeth in the area as represented on the stone cast (Fig. 8-17). The denture tooth and the acrylic saddle are removed from the framework by carefully cutting away the retention from the tissue side, and by removing the acrylic from around the attachments. The objective is to retain as much of the original outer contour of the saddle as possible. Later, using this plaster index, the denture tooth and saddle can be accurately related to the framework, the case invested by normal means, and the new acrylic processed in the tissue area (Fig. 8-18).
3. The new occlusal rest is waxed on the stone cast (Fig. 8-19).
4. The new part and the partial denture framework are related on the refractory cast and welded by electrosoldering. Some laboratories will use normal precious-metal, low-fus-

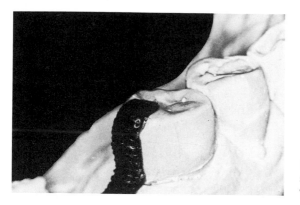

Fig. 8-19 Typical waxup of new occlusal rest, with strut included. This new casting would normally be welded to the framework at the gingival end.

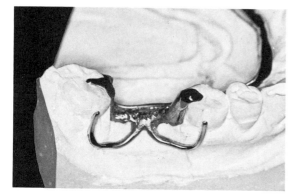

Fig. 8-20a Partial denture on stone cast after electrowelding of new occlusal rest and strut to framework.

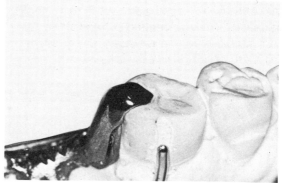

Fig. 8-20b Closer view showing that, in this case, a new strut was waxed over the old one to result in a better welded joint. This option is preferred when there is room for it.

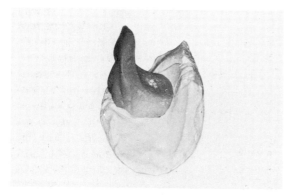

Fig. 8-21 Acrylic tooth luted to a plaster index, ready for refitting to the cast and attachment to the partial denture framework.

ing solder. However, if the particular laboratory is so equipped, the electrosoldering method is superior for chrome-cobalt-type partial denture frameworks. It has been shown that electro-soldering can produce a joint with a tensile strength as great as that of cast metal.[7]

5. The soldered framework is tried on the stone cast and its fit evaluated for accuracy (Figs. 8-20a and b).

6. After electrosoldering, the denture tooth along with the acrylic saddle is reattached with new acrylic to the framework (Fig. 8-21).

7. The case is returned to the dentist.

Step 8

Try in the corrected partial denture, *making certain above all that the framework fits all other attachments exactly as before.* Do not concentrate too much on the new occlusal rest or assume that if it seats properly, all is well. In fact, the new rest may seat properly even though other parts of the framework are now unserviceable owing to distortion in the laboratory, or to imperfect seating in the impression before pouring the cast.

Step 9

Check the occlusion, on both the new occlusal rest and the replaced adjacent denture tooth. Because the tissue-bearing surface of the adjacent saddle was also replaced, check and adjust it as with any new acrylic tissue surface.

Replacement of a broken clasp

One of the more commonly required corrections to partial dentures is the replacement of a broken cast metal clasp. A clasp can fail for the following reasons:

1. Too many attempts to adjust the clasp. Particularly with chrome-cobalt frameworks, there is a limit to the number of times a clasp arm can be safely bent before the adverse effects of work hardening come into play.
2. Original casting was too thin to endure long-term stress. Remember that the clasp bends every time the partial denture is placed or removed.
3. Occasionally a clasp is broken off when the denture is dropped or when a patient attempts to adjust it.

Replacing a broken clasp is done principally by the laboratory technician. The dentist makes an adequate impression and evaluates the denture while he or she has access to the patient, an advantage the technician does not have.

Method

In this method, a clasp is replaced with a new casting of the same type of alloy as the original partial denture casting. A separate technique is described later for adding a new clasp to an existing partial denture where none was present in the original design.

Step 1

Place the partial denture in the mouth and check the fit of all attachments, paying particular attention to whether the denture is stable without the clasp. It may not be stable when placed under occlusal load, but it must be stable enough to maintain perfect position during the impression procedure.

Step 2

With the denture in place, carefully examine the area of failure, bearing in mind that the more preparation of the immediate area that can be done by the dentist, the better.

The following can be done prior to making the impression and sending the case to the laboratory:

1. Generally, the clasp will be broken at its weakest point, thus leaving a very small cross-sectional area for welding on a new clasp (Fig. 8-22). It is always best to grind away the rest of the clasp-arm all the way back to the point at which it originates from the shoulder of the attachment (Fig. 8-23). With sufficient reduction of the clasp-arm, a larger interface is available for the welding operation, and a greater degree of freedom is afforded in waxing the new clasp-arm. In this regard it will often be necessary to replace the entire attachment, including the rest. This is more often the case in circumferential clasps, whereas I bar clasps attach to the major connector through the acrylic retention rather than to the direct retainer. That is why this step is so important. Were the impression to be made with the rest of the

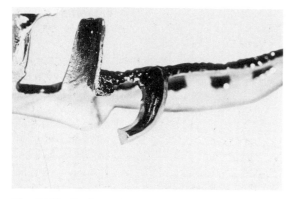

Fig. 8-22 Broken clasp-arm without a sufficiently large cross-section for proper electrowelding.

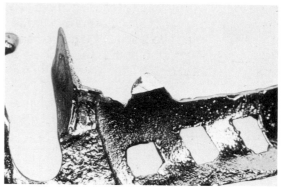

Fig. 8-23 Clasp-arm trimmed back to a point where there is an adequate cross-sectional area.

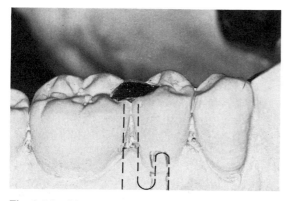

Fig. 8-24 Clasp-arm broken off at the point where it was attached to the occlusal rest between premolar and molar. Obviously, it was too thin from lack of tooth preparation to provide adequate strength. Dotted line shows position of original clasp-arm.

attachment in place, and the technician to later decide that it would be best to replace the entire attachment, the area under the remainder of the attachment would not be accurate or neat enough for the technician to use in waxing the new part.

2. The tooth may need to be modified to provide more occlusal clearance if the clasp-arm originates from the occlusal rest. It is often found in this situation that insufficient reduction existed, since often the opposing cusp fits into the embrasure and limits the space (Fig. 8-24).

3. The tooth may need to be modified to provide better retention than before. This is a

golden opportunity to significantly improve the restoration. Since a whole new clasp-arm will be waxed to the contour given to the technician on the stone cast, why not be certain that the contour exhibits the best possible retentive features?

Step 3

Make a full-arch irreversible hydrocolloid impression with the partial denture in place and accurately reproduce the tooth area to be in contact with the new clasp. Use a thinner-than-normal mix of alginate to reduce the risk of any displacement of the impression caused by pressure from the material while the tray is going into position. Occasionally, it will be necessary to stabilize the framework temporarily with a self-curing resin, connecting the partial denture framework to one or more teeth (Fig. 8-3).

Step 4

Remove this full-arch impression. Usually, the partial denture will be removed with the impression and will remain in perfect position, ready for pouring of the cast. However, if the partial denture does remain in the mouth, the dentist rather than the technician should take responsibility for placing it correctly into the impression. Occasionally, it will be necessary to remove small areas of alginate that interfere with clasp areas in order to place the partial denture back into the impression. This is of little concern, because this impression only requires that the denture be completely seated into it when it is poured and that the immediate area of the correction be a perfect reproduction of the situation in the mouth.

Make a second irreversible alginate impression of the area of the correction, without the partial denture in place. This impression can be in a simple quadrant tray and will be used to make the wax pattern in some cases (Fig. 8-16).

If the laboratory is nearby, send the impressions there for pouring, as it is usually best to have the technician who will ultimately be responsible for waxing and assembling the case also pour the impression. However, if this arrangement is not possible, the dentist should pour the cast in a densite stone. When pouring this impression, consider the following points:

1. Use a standard blockout wax to block out any undercuts in the acrylic saddle areas, except for any saddle adjacent to the area where the new clasp will be welded to the partial denture. This acrylic will need to be removed anyway, and when it is replaced it will be important that the cast accurately reproduces the contour of the patient's ridge.
2. Reinforce any abutment teeth which, in the judgment of the operator, could be broken off when the partial denture is removed from the stone cast. This can be done by simply placing a brass dowel pin or a stiff wire into the impression of the tooth in question prior to pouring the stone cast.
3. Lightly lubricate the tissue surface of the acrylic saddles with a tin foil substitute so the stone will not adhere.

Step 5

The following procedure is performed by the laboratory technician:

1. The partial denture is removed from the cast and a refractory cast is made to be used later in the welding operation.
2. If the clasp is adjacent to an area of acrylic, an occlusal index is made in plaster that will

relate the denture tooth to the remainder of the teeth in the area represented on the stone cast (Fig. 8-18).
3. The denture tooth or teeth and the acrylic saddle are removed from the framework by carefully cutting away the retention from the tissue side and by removing the acrylic from around the attachments. The object of this procedure is to retain as much of the original outer contour of the saddle as possible. Later, using the plaster index just referred to in the previous step, the denture tooth and saddle can be related accurately to the framework, the case invested by normal means, and new acrylic processed in the tissue area.
4. The new clasp-arm, or entire attachment as the case may be, is waxed on the stone cast as would be done for a new occlusal rest.
5. The new clasp-arm is then cast in the same alloy as the denture. On occasion, the technician will prefer to wax the new part on the separate cast mentioned earlier.
6. The new part is related on the refractory cast and welded using an electrosoldering method. Some laboratories will use normal precious-metal, low-fusing solder. However, if the particular laboratory is equipped to do it, the electrosoldering method is superior for chrome-cobalt type of partial denture frameworks. It has been shown that electrosoldering can produce a joint with a tensile strength as great as that of cast metal.[7]
7. The soldered framework is tried on the stone cast to verify the fit.
8. After electrosoldering, the denture tooth or teeth and the acrylic saddle are reattached with new acrylic to the framework (Fig. 8-21).
9. The case is returned to the dentist.

Step 6

The dentist will now try in the corrected partial denture making certain, above all else that the framework fits all of the other attachments exactly as it did before. It is easy at this point to concentrate one's attention unduly on the new clasp-arm or attachment and think that if it fits properly, all is well. However, the new clasp might fit fine even though other parts of the framework are now unserviceable due to distortion in the laboratory, or to imperfect seating in the impression before pouring the cast.

Step 7

Check the adaptation to the tissue of any acrylic saddles that were replaced in the laboratory, as you would with any new denture, and verify that the occlusion is also correct, particularly where saddle areas were removed and replaced.

Addition of a retentive clasp-arm

It sometimes is necessary to attach a retentive clasp-arm to a removable partial denture where none was placed in the original design. The following are some situations which would indicate the need for this procedure:

1. An abutment tooth is lost, which also creates the need for other modifications to the partial denture, such as adding a tooth on the denture to replace the missing abutment, or placing a new saddle in this area. This will be addressed later in this chapter.
2. More retention is needed than was provided for in the original design. The advisability of performing this procedure will be largely determined by the presence of a lingual plate or arm in the original casting to provide the needed reciprocation for the new retentive arm. If reciprocation is absent use the procedure for replacement of the entire cast attachment, including rest, guiding planes, and reciprocating surface.
3. A broken cast clasp needs to be replaced with another clasp, and a cast clasp is inadvisable for one reason or another. This method is preferred by many for replacing any clasp.

The procedure essentially involves forming a wrought wire clasp on a cast, then attaching it into the acrylic flange of the existing partial denture. This technique differs from other corrections in that it is neither necessary, nor advisable to remove the partial denture from the stone cast before completing the attachment of the clasp. The denture is best left in place on the cast until it is time to polish the corrected area.

Techniques presented in dental literature involve such variations as adding an IC attachment to the partial denture and modifying the tooth to receive it,[8] or casting a new clasp to be attached to the partial denture. These new clasps can be retained either by soldering to the framework,[9] or by processing a new acrylic resin base to the new clasp.[10]

Method

Step 1

Determine that the other attachments of the partial denture fit and that the denture is stable in the mouth as with all techniques presented here involving the replacement of all or part of an attachment. In the present situation, it is assumed that the original occlusal or incisal rest which was part of this attachment is still present and seats properly. If this is untrue, as in the case of a lost abutment tooth, then include a new rest in the replacement and employ the procedure described later in this chapter. The partial denture framework should have the same degree of stability as before, though it would have less retention if a retentive clasp arm is missing. This method replaces only the arm, not the entire attachment.

Step 2

Make an impression with the partial denture in place in the mouth. It may be necessary temporarily to hold it in place by applying a small amount of self-curing acrylic, sticky wax, or compound to the attachment involved and the adjacent tooth, since the retention in this area is missing. Use a thinner than normal mix of alginate to reduce the risk that the partial denture will be displaced from the pressure of the material while the tray is going into position (Fig. 8-3).

Step 3

Pour the impression in dental stone with the partial denture in place, taking the following precautions:

1. With a standard blockout wax, block out any undercuts in the acrylic saddles. As opposed to some other corrective procedures in this text, all saddles will remain on the partial denture in this procedure and therefore must have their undercuts blocked out.
2. Lightly lubricate the tissue surface of the acrylic saddles with a tin-foil substitute so the stone will not adhere.

Step 4

Since in some cases the surface to be engaged by the clasp was not originally used for retention, it is best to survey a diagnostic cast made without the partial denture in place, as described later in this chapter. This is one way to confirm that the new clasp-arm will provide the predicted retention before embarking on the modification of the partial denture.

Step 5

Since the occlusal rest is already present in most cases, and the only addition will be on an axial surface, it will not be necessary to make and mount an opposing cast.

Step 6

As will be seen in a later step, the new clasp will be retained in the partial denture by embedding it in the existing acrylic flange on the side *opposite* to the side of the tooth into which the retentive clasp will engage, either facially or lingually. This presupposes a circumferential design, the usual use for a wrought wire clasp. The wire embedded in the acrylic on the opposite side of the tooth allows the retentive arm to approach the undercut from the occlusal aspect, thereby crossing the survey line. The reciprocation is derived from the part of the wrought wire on the side of the tooth where the wire is embedded in

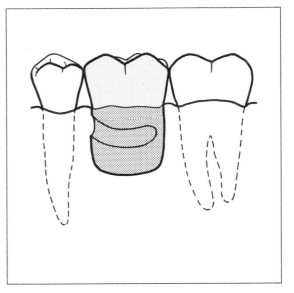

Fig. 8-25   Groove in lingual flange.

the acrylic saddle, and therefore, a groove must be cut in the facial or lingual flange. The exact location, length, and depth of the groove will vary depending on the case. Basically, one should attempt to make a curved groove at least 6 or 7 mm long, and as deep as possible without perforating the tissue side of the saddle. The curve acts as resistance to wire rotation (Fig. 8-25). This can be accomplished without removing the partial denture from the cast.[11]

Step 7

Mark the survey line on the cast which has the partial denture in place transferring the orientation from the diagnostic cast to the working cast with the partial denture in place. Draw the survey line on the involved surface.

Step 8

Form the new clasp from a piece of 18-gauge wrought wire following the survey line for proper position into the undercut. Form the other end of the wire to fit into the groove in the flange of the partial denture. Round the free end of the new clasp-arm.

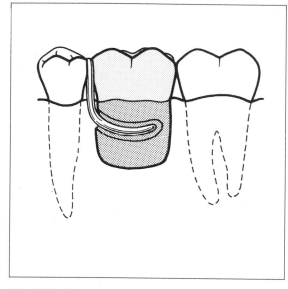

Fig. 8-26 Facial view showing new retentive clasp.

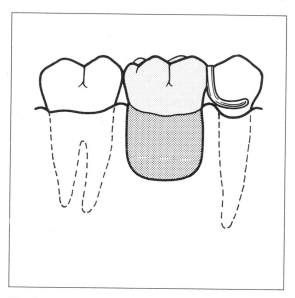

Fig. 8-27 Wire seated in groove ready for the addition of self-curing acrylic resin. Note curve in wire to limit rotation after acrylic is set.

Step 9

Lute the new wrought wire clasp-arm to the involved surface of the abutment tooth on the stone cast (Fig. 8-26), and simultaneously ensure that the other end of the wire fits into the bottom of the groove (Fig. 8-27). Wet the old acrylic in the depth of the groove with monomer and carefully flow a creamy mixture of self-curing tissue-colored acrylic into the groove around the wire. Add acrylic sufficient to make the new material slightly higher than the surrounding flange surface, to allow for finishing.

Step 10

Remove the partial denture from the cast, being careful not to distort the framework, and smooth the added acrylic to the level of the surrounding flange surface. Polish as with any new denture.

Correction of fractured acrylic resin base

When acrylic resin bases become fractured, it is most commonly a complete fracture caused by the denture being dropped. We are not concerned in this discussion about the mending of a fracture which has occurred while the denture was in function in the mouth, as this type of failure is usually traceable to problems of space and thickness of materials inherent in the original design of the prosthesis. These types of failures usually call for construction of a new partial denture that does not incorporate the errors in design of the previous denture (Fig. 8-28).

Generally these corrections are done with self-curing methylmethacrylate resin without flasking. The advantages of this method are discussed in the section on relining partial dentures, pages 180 to 183. It bears emphasizing that there is a certain degree of risk involved anytime a completed partial denture is reflasked and then later broken out of the flask. It is always advisable to avoid this procedure if at all possible.

One important criterion is that the separate parts must index together in perfect relationship. Consider the process by which the denture was originally constructed. The framework was related to a full-arch cast, and the saddles were then waxed to the cast according to this relationship. A successful result will be unlikely if the two parts cannot be indexed well together at this point, since there is no longer a cast to use. Also, the parts cannot be related well in the mouth since one of the fragments would be relying on the support of the soft tissue for indexing, which is not accurate enough. In the rare case that this was the chosen method, relining would be required after the correction. Rebasing—simply replacing all of the acrylic at one time—may be the better treatment to follow.

It is axiomatic that many times there is a certain amount of pressure exerted on either the dentist, technician, or both, to expedite a correction procedure so that a patient will be without the denture for the shortest possible time. This often results in the abuse of the self-curing acrylic, which may result in either a weak or a distorted result. Since it is a chemical reaction, the time allowed for completely curing the resin has a direct effect on the strength and dimensional stability of the correction. It has been said that the self-curing resin can have greater dimensional stability than heat-cured resins, though the latter will usually be more resistant to stains or color changes caused by greater surface density. The most important consideration in this technique, however, is dimensional stability, which is best attained by leaving the correction to cure for 2 or 3 hours rather than the minimal time of 20 to 30 minutes, as is often done. Longer curing results in more complete polymerization and a more satisfactory long-term result.[12]

Method

Step 1

The dentist should ascertain from careful inspection of the denture and the broken part, whether the unbroken acrylic material is usable and in good condition. Try the denture in the mouth and verify that, except for the broken

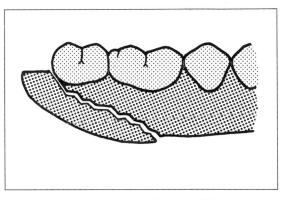

Fig. 8-28 Typical fracture of a partial denture base in which parts can be related well and the attachment to the metal framework is not involved.

segment, it satisfies all of the generally accepted criteria. Outside the mouth, ascertain that the parts index perfectly and without perceptible movement. Use of the stereomicroscope is very helpful in making this determination.

The following steps for the actual mending of the parts can be performed by either the laboratory or the dentist.

Step 2

Attach the two parts together with sticky wax and wooden sticks as needed, confining this procedure to the outer surfaces that will not contact the tissue (Fig. 8-29).

Lightly lubricate the tissue surface of the acrylic saddles with petroleum jelly or tin-foil substitute.

Step 3

Pour a cast of the tissue surface of the saddle, including the broken segment, in dental stone mixed with slurry water to hasten the set. This stone cast is the key to making an accurate correction, and it must contact enough of both parts to provide stable positioning of the two segments after the sticky wax and sticks are removed. Lute the two parts securely to the stone cast.

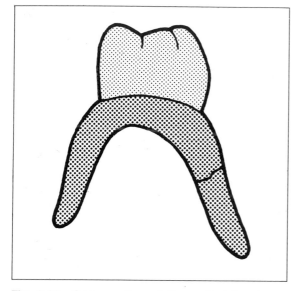

Fig. 8-29 Cross-section of flange that has been related correctly, indicating no change in the tissue surface.

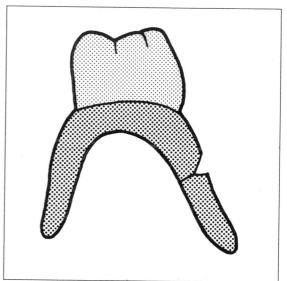

Fig. 8-30 V-shaped notch in outer surface of the flange, not so deep as to involve the tissue surface.

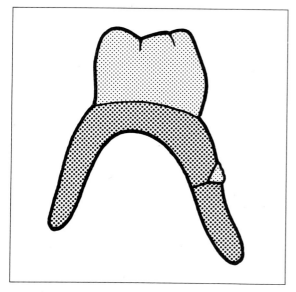

Fig. 8-31 New acrylic added to partial denture showing the areas of contact between the new acrylic and the two parts of the partial denture flange.

Step 4

After removing the sticky wax, cut a V-shaped notch in the junction of the two segments without penetrating the tissue surface of the saddle. The two sides of the V should be at 45- to 90-degree angles to each other. Determine whether there is enough surface area exposed on both parts to effect adequate bonding with the new acrylic material. If there is not, rule out this technique and do a rebase (Fig. 8-30).

Step 5

The best method for adding the new material is to sprinkle on the polymer after wetting the involved surfaces of the old segments with monomer dispensed from a small eye dropper. Do not allow the monomer to spread onto the outer surface, because this can be damaging if the original material was not one of the newer cross-linked types. Sprinkle on the polymer and repeat this process until the notch has been slightly overfilled (Fig. 8-31).

Step 6

Place the assembly in the pressure pot under

warm water and allow it to cure completely, usually for 2 to 3 hours. Some patients will demonstrate a reaction to the self-curing methylmethacrylate. Though rare, reactions occur often enough to justify the practice of attaining a more complete cure by using the pressure pot. In some cases, the only solution will be to use a heat-cured material and go through the flasking process just as with a new denture.

Step 7

Remove the assembly from the pressure pot and the saddle from the stone cast. Inspect the tissue side of the saddle under the stereomicroscope to ascertain that the joint on the tissue surface fits perfectly. If it does not, the partial denture will probably need to be relined, so initiate this procedure at the seating appointment, without delay. If the joint fits perfectly, smooth the new material to the level of the surrounding old acrylic and polish it.

Replacement of denture teeth

As with saddle area fractures, replacing denture teeth is needed when a denture has been dropped. If a denture tooth is lost during function in the mouth, a simple replacement of the denture tooth will seldom suffice. This is because when such a tooth is loosened in normal function, it usually is due to a lack of retention for the tooth in the original design. The method of replacement depends on the original retention method of the denture tooth and the material from which the tooth is made, as follows:

1. Most denture teeth are made of acrylic and are held onto partial dentures by bonding with the acrylic which also makes up the saddle.
2. Occasionally porcelain teeth are used, in which case retention is mechanical, usually by means of a hole (diatoric) in the porcelain tooth into which the acrylic of the saddle is forced upon flasking, or the use of pins.

3. A third less common retention method uses tube teeth pontics. The framework is cast with posts that are then used to retain porcelain denture teeth by fitting into holes along the long axis of the teeth. A cementing medium of some type must also be used.

Since denture teeth are most commonly made of acrylic, the method described here is for replacement of an acrylic tooth that has become dislodged from the denture. Even with lost porcelain denture teeth, the technique for placing an acrylic tooth into the existing denture has advantages. With the great improvement in the quality and esthetics of the acrylic teeth, however, there is little justification for using porcelain teeth in dentures now, especially in light of the attendant disadvantage of adverse wear to opposing teeth.

Method

Step 1

Remove the remainder of the old tooth, usually by grinding down to the base acrylic. When the tooth has detached from the base material completely intact, simply reuse the entire original tooth.

Step 2

Select an appropriate replacement acrylic tooth, paying particular attention to shade and facial contour. If a compromise is needed in the duplication of the old tooth, it should be done on the lingual rather than the facial surface. For example if one tooth is the correct length for the facial, but too short on the lingual, select it rather than one with the opposite characteristics. In this manner, any acrylic which is added to take up the space will not be on the facial surface where it would be seen.

Step 3

Adjust the replacement acrylic tooth to fit into

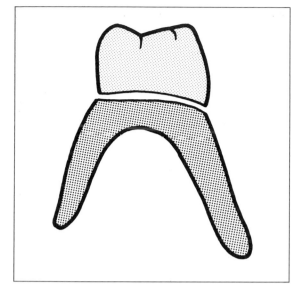

Fig. 8-32 New tooth in position, showing space to be occupied by new acrylic resin.

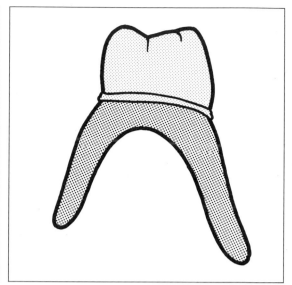

Fig. 8-33 Self-curing acrylic resin in place, attaching new tooth to partial denture base.

the recess previously occupied by the now missing tooth (Fig. 8-32). Temporarily attach the new tooth to the partial denture with sticky wax on the lingual surface, and evaluate the facial contour, the alignment, and the occlusion.

Step 4

Make the actual attachment of the tooth to the denture with self-curing acrylic resin in one of the following two ways:

1. If the fit of the tooth on the facial at the gingival line is essentially correct, requiring but a small amount of fill-in with new material, flow a relatively thin mix of self-curing acrylic into the space on both the facial and the lingual surfaces. The acrylic can be either tooth colored or tissue colored, depending on the need in that situation (Fig. 8-33).
2. If 1 mm or more of material is to be added, then follow a more involved procedure of waxing in the missing contour, and making a plaster matrix of the surface of the new tooth and the adjacent teeth. This matrix should cover the facial of the tooth, most of the

occlusal or incisal surface, and a few millimeters of the gingival denture base on the facial surface. Use fast-setting plaster to hasten the set. The matrix need not be removable. Boil out the wax after removing the new tooth. After wetting both the tooth and the denture base with monomer, mix a small amount of self-curing acrylic, usually tooth colored, and place it into the recess. Seat the new acrylic tooth into position and then place in a pressure pot for 2 or 3 hours if possible, contour, and finish.

Addition of a tooth to a partial denture to replace a lost natural tooth

The lost natural tooth may be totally unrelated to the partial denture, or it may have been an abutment tooth. Most likely it was lost because of uncontrolled periodontal disease. As an abutment it may have provided retention, an occlusal rest, or guiding planes. If so, the best treatment is seldom to add the former abutment tooth to the partial denture. The reason for this is that when the denture was first designed, the tooth in question was deemed to be an essential feature of the design as an abutment tooth. It is unlikely that the denture would be able to function the same way without it as an abutment.

Most instances of lost abutment teeth will require the construction of a new partial denture. Take this fact into account from a preventive standpoint, and be realistic when determining whether a particular compromised tooth should be used as an abutment in the initial planning of the partial denture. The one exception to this principle occurs when the tooth was a terminal abutment, in which case a tooth-borne partial denture can sometimes be converted to a distal-extension one. Even so, it is most often advisable to construct a new partial denture, since the original design probably did not provide for attachments on the other abutment teeth that are compatible with a distal-extension design. The conversion of a tooth-borne to a distal-extension denture is a common error that results in adverse forces on the remaining abutment teeth, and should be done only in compelling situations, or where this possibility was taken into account in the design of the original partial denture.

Unlike the other modifications discussed in this chapter, adding a tooth to a partial denture often requires addition of a new acrylic retention to the framework casting. Although this may not seem difficult, it is often a complicated procedure. It might be helpful to consider a couple of typical situations which arise in this regard:

New tooth remote from framework

When no part of the framework is anywhere near the new edentulous area, three possible procedures can be followed:

1. If possible, replace the missing tooth with a fixed bridge and do not involve the partial denture at all. It is also important in such a case to question whether a mouth that has already lost some teeth years before, and has recently lost another, is an appropriate fixed bridge candidate from a periodontal standpoint.
2. Modify the metal casting to achieve acrylic retention in the newly edentulous area.
3. Make a new partial denture with a framework designed from the outset to include the newly edentulous area.

New tooth close to framework

If the lost tooth was not an abutment, but did have the metal casting in intimate relationship to it, a guiding plane, lingual plate, or border of the casting may be adjacent to the gingival crest/tooth junction. If so, it may be possible to mechanically add acrylic to the framework and thereby replace the missing tooth. However, the original waxup in this area may not have been done with the intention of ever attaching a new section to it for acrylic retention. Indeed it may be impossible, depending on the bulk of metal available to work with, as well as other unanticipated factors such as the occlusion.

Of all the modifications made to existing partial dentures, adding acrylic to the original framework to replace a lost tooth is the most difficult and the most prone to failure, a fact that must be made clear to the patient prior to attempting to do so. When considering the advisability of this alteration to an existing partial denture, it is essential to recognize that virtually all of the factors involved in designing a new partial denture must be taken into account. When an abutment tooth is lost, we must acknowledge that a design with different parameters than the original one exists. Some of these differences can be:

1. The span of the saddle is now at least one tooth longer—more if this was an isolated abutment with an edentulous space on each side.
2. The new abutment tooth which replaces the old one may not be as sound periodontally or functionally.
3. Depending on the location of other abutment teeth, it might be better to change the

entire design rather than make this one alteration.

There will always be a need for a reline procedure on this new saddle after a period of time for healing of the new extraction site. This should be made clear to the patient and carefully considered during the design of the correction.

Finally, accept that this procedure is seldom the appropriate permanent treatment. *However, it can often be useful as a temporary expedient until the ridge is remodeled and a new partial denture made.*

Method: Added retention for new acrylic

Step 1

Extract any remaining portions of the missing tooth, keeping the following in mind:

1. Take extra care when trimming the bone to verify that the areas remaining will not irritate the soft tissue during healing, since there will be a partial denture saddle placed immediately.
2. If possible, the tissue should be sutured to attain primary closure of the socket, providing this will not cause abnormal bone healing. This will often result in a more controlled modeling of the bone, possibly in combination with a temporary (or treatment) partial denture.

Step 2

Make an overimpression in irreversible hydrocolloid with the denture in place, taking several factors into account:

1. The stability of the partial denture may present a problem if the extracted tooth was a critical abutment. The denture may need to be temporarily stabilized with a small amount of self-curing acrylic, compound, or even acid-etched composite, by attaching strate-

gic clasp arms or occlusal rests to adjacent tooth structure. The method and material can vary with the situation, as long as the partial denture does not move during the seating of the impression tray (Fig. 8-3).
2. Before making the impression, carefully examine the partial denture and modify it as necessary to eliminate any area of the existing metal framework adjacent to the new edentulous area that could interfere with a perfect tissue impression.
3. The impression should have as ideal extension as possible, since in most of these cases there will not be the usual opportunity for picking up the extensions in an altered cast impression.

Step 3

The laboratory is responsible for the following nine procedures, so they are described here only briefly:

1. The technician blocks out any undercuts in the partial and then lubricates the tissue side of the saddles. The stone cast is poured into the impression with the partial in place to develop a master cast. As usual, any teeth likely to fracture when removing the partial from the cast are reinforced.
2. The partial denture is removed from the cast and the metal at the junction area is prepared to receive the new cast section and later the acrylic. Any number of adjustments may be made to the metal casting to allow a successful soldering procedure, most of which will be aimed at developing as large a cross-section as possible. A chamfered, hollow-ground finish line should be developed so that a thin flash of the new resin will not result. This is usually done in the old casting, adjacent to the solder joint, but occasionally it can be done in the new casting itself, depending on the situation.
3. With the partial denture in place on the stone cast, undercuts are blocked out and a refractory cast developed.

4. The retention for acrylic is waxed on the refractory cast.
5. The new section is cast in the same alloy as the original framework.
6. The new casting is cleaned and fit to the master stone cast, which has the partial denture in place. It is most important that the joint area to be soldered has sufficient space for a good result, but not so much as to complicate the procedure. Ideally, the space should be no more than 1 mm. It has been shown that very strong joints can be made by electrosoldering to vitallium and similar alloys when the space between parts is as small as .25 mm.[13]
7. The parts are electrosoldered directly on the stone cast.
8. With the modified partial denture still on the stone cast and the cast mounted in occlusion with the opposing cast on an articulator, the teeth are set and the saddle waxup completed according to the predetermined outline. The dentist is responsible for the extensions. This determination should not be left to the technician.
9. The partial denture is flasked, processed, and finished. While the other saddle areas are in acrylic rather than wax during investing they should be treated as new acrylic after breaking them out of the plaster.

Step 4

Try in the partial denture, adjust the occlusion, and check the tissue surface of the new saddle with indicator paste. Also, remove any sutures, if used, during this appointment.

Step 5

The most significant difference between this insertion procedure and that of a new partial denture is awareness that a reline will be needed after a period of time and that the fit may be less than ideal until then.

Method: Retention in the existing framework casting

Use this method when there is no need for new acrylic retention to be added to the partial framework and when retention for the replacement tooth and a relatively small saddle can be developed in the existing framework casting.

Step 1

Extract the failing tooth, keeping in mind the following:

A little extra care should be taken in trimming the bone to ensure that the remaining areas will not irritate the soft tissue during healing, since there will be a partial denture saddle placed immediately.

If possible, the tissue should be sutured to attain primary closure of the socket, providing this will not cause abnormal bone healing. This will often result in a more controlled modeling of the bone, possibly in combination with a temporary, or treatment, partial denture.

Step 2

Make an overimpression with the partial denture in place using an irreversible hydrocolloid material (Fig. 8-3). Prior to this, examine the partial denture casting in the area of the missing tooth, and remove any metal from the casting that could interfere with making a perfect impression of the ridge tissue. Do not remove metal from the framework that will be needed later for retention of the new tooth.

Step 3

Pour the stone into the impression with the partial denture in place to make a master cast. Reinforce any teeth prone to fracture when the partial is later removed. Block out any undercuts in acrylic saddle areas. Lubricate such areas with petroleum jelly. Remove the partial denture from the stone cast.

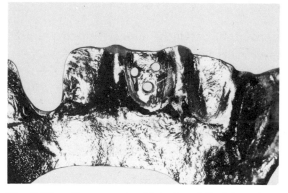

Fig. 8-34a Framework with holes drilled for retention of a new acrylic resin tooth, viewed from the facial aspect.

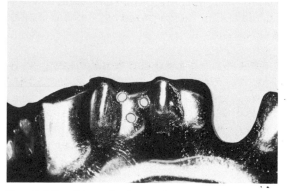

Fig. 8-34b Lingual view prior to countersinking holes.

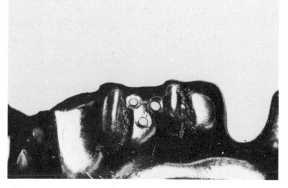

Fig. 8-34c Holes countersunk for retention of acrylic resin, which will attach the pontic to the partial denture framework.

Step 4

Develop retention for new acrylic in the metal casting by drilling holes in guiding planes and lingual plates. If the holes are located on opposing surfaces, they need not always penetrate to the finished surface of the casting. For example, several shallow holes made into the areas of opposing plates which were previously on the mesial and distal surfaces of the lost tooth will often afford adequate retention. Opposing surfaces are often unavailable, so you will often need to drill the holes through the plate of the framework casting. Countersink the holes on the outer surface for retention of the self-curing acrylic resin (Figs. 8-34a to c).

Step 5

Usually it is better to make the replacement of a small tooth by adjusting the new acrylic replacement tooth to fit the space and clear the ridge by 1 to 2 mm, then lute it into position with tissue-colored, self-curing acrylic resin. This presupposes that ridge coverage is not being done over a large area. If a saddle with a large flange is being made as part of this correction, then flask the partial denture and process according to normal practice. Finish the partial denture and insert, making adjustments for occlusion and tissue contact.

Conversion of partial denture to interim full denture

Although a full-denture prosthesis implies the ultimate failure of treatment, the patient at "the end of the road" can benefit from wearing an existing partial denture as an interim full prosthesis during healing after a final extraction.

Interim full dentures also have psychological advantages for patients. The change from a partial to a full denture is a major transition in the patient's life. A modified existing partial denture, which the patient is accustomed to and likely quite satisfied with, can be a very useful crutch until the final full denture is constructed. The advantages of this procedure are discussed by Payne.[14] Techniques such as those advocated by Bailey[15] and Abbott[16] emphasize making the alteration as simply as possible. Any technique for an interim full denture prosthesis must satisfy the following criteria:

1. Promote good healing of the recent extraction sockets.
2. Attain the function of a full denture (retention and stability) and simultaneously make the interim restoration feel like the existing one.
3. Make the modification as expeditiously as possible.

Method

Step 1

Make an overimpression with irreversible hydrocolloid material with the existing partial denture in place, noting the following:

1. If a terminal abutment tooth is to be extracted, remove the attachment, unless it is needed to help permanently retain the replacement plastic denture tooth. This decision must therefore be made in each individual case.
2. Stabilize the partial, with denture adhesive, if needed.
3. Use a thin mix of impression material to keep the partial denture from moving during the procedure.

Step 2

Since the new acrylic will be attached to the existing acrylic, the latter should be beveled or feathered to allow for a sufficiently large attachment area for the new temporary resin.

Step 3

Lubricate the cast in the area of the addition with tin-foil substitute. Replace the partial denture on the cast. If a maxillary, cut a postdam into the cast. For either a maxillary or a mandibular, outline the desired extension on the stone model. Wet the junction area of the existing partial denture acrylic with monomer, then sprinkle on a new acrylic section as done for constructing an orthodontic appliance.

Step 4

When this has completely cured, in about 2 to 3 hours, perform a reline procedure. Refer to the section on relining of partial dentures for this procedure. The reline procedure accomplishes several things:

1. Adaptation to the entire tissue-bearing area is better than if the corrected section contacts the tissue.
2. The reline acrylic strengthens the junction between old and new sections.
3. Problems with tissue irritation caused by monomer are minimized by heat-cured acrylic contacting the tissue.

Step 5

It will sometimes be advisable to place a tissue-conditioning material instead of relining the corrected partial denture with acrylic. This judgment must be made by the dentist, and will take into consideration such things as tissue health and tone. Tissue-conditioning material is advantageous because it can be periodically changed as the extraction site heals.

Step 6

The insertion procedures are the same as for any relined full denture or denture with tissue conditioner.

Relining partial dentures

Relining the acrylic saddles of a partial denture may be necessary because of resorption of the edentulous ridge while the denture has been in service. If a distal extension saddle, there will usually be a change in the stability of the restoration, often noticed by the patient, but sometimes not. If the saddle is tooth borne, then the primary complaint will often be that food gets under the saddle.

It eventually will be necessary to reline the saddle after healing and bone modeling in cases where a denture was placed very soon after tooth extraction. Relining a brand new partial denture may also be necessary if an error was made during either processing the saddle or construction of an altered cast.

The reline procedure involves creating an adequate space for impression material in the original saddle, making an impression using the denture as a tray, and processing new acrylic to the tissue surface of the saddle. With a short-span, tooth-borne saddle, a direct reline material is more than expedient—it is often preferred since it does not involve flasking and deflasking the partial framework and the attendant dangers of those procedures. Consider the material comprising the construction of the dental base. If the denture is relatively old, it is probably made of a non-cross-linked acrylic. Do not use the direct reline materials with these acrylics, because crazing or distortion can be caused by the monomer. However, modern cross-linked resins are not subject to this effect to any great degree.[11]

When deciding whether to reline a partial denture saddle, consider also the condition of the periphery. A well-made saddle has a satisfactory peripheral seal, even though the tissue-bearing area needs relining, because most of the resorption on the ridge is in the area of alveolar bone. It is hoped that the peripheral seal is extended farther onto the basal bone.

Dental literature addresses the methods for determining the need for a reline[17] a rebase,[18] and the methods for making these alterations.[19,20,14]

Method: Direct reline method

Step 1

Relieve the tissue side of the saddle in question enough to allow adequate thickness, about 2 mm, of the reline material. Extend this relief onto the curvature of the periphery of the flange and end outside the tissue contact area, but not so far as to significantly change the length of the flange (Fig. 8-35).

This provides a junction of the new and old materials that is not in direct contact with the ridge tissue, and it assures that pressure is not exerted on the ridge tissue as the new material is being placed.

Step 2

Apply a thin coat of petroleum jelly to the external surfaces in order to make cleanup and polishing easier. Mix the material according to the manufacturer's directions, and wet the relieved surface of the old acrylic saddle with new monomer to aid bonding.

Step 3

After the material has attained body, apply it to the saddle and seat the partial denture in the mouth. The new material, which does flow onto the periphery, should be border molded as with any denture impression. Verify that the occlusal rests adjacent to the saddle are perfectly seated and that there is no new reline material under them. The patient should close into CO while the material sets. If upon examination under a microscope there is any new acrylic material under the rests, the framework is not seated properly and the entire process must be repeated. An improperly seated framework is a considerably greater defect than the original indication for relining, which was simply poor tissue adaptation.

Step 4

After the material has set, remove the denture

and trim the material at the periphery according to the manufacturer's instructions.

Method: Indirect reline method

Step 1

Relieve the tissue side of the partial denture saddle an adequate amount to allow for approximately 1.0 to 1.5 mm of impression material. Extend this relief onto the curvature of the periphery of the flange and end it outside the tissue contact area, but not so far as to significantly change the length of the flange. This provides a junction of the new and old materials that is not in direct contact with the ridge tissue, and it assures that pressure is not exerted on the ridge tissue as the impression material is being placed (Fig. 8-35).

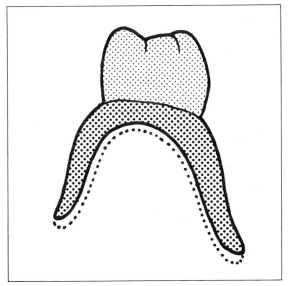

Fig. 8-35 The dotted line represents the acrylic relieved from the tissue surface of the partial denture saddle to make room for impression material, and ultimately for the new acrylic resin, in the case of a reline.

Step 2

Make an impression of the ridge using the partial denture saddle as a custom tray. Use either a static or a functional technique to generate the impression.

Static method—Use any light or medium body impression material of the elastomeric family or a metallic oxide paste. Do not use heavy body material that will cause tissue compression. Apply the proper adhesive, being sure that the adhesive extends onto the facial and lingual saddle surfaces for good adaptation and retention of the impression material at the periphery. Apply the impression material conservatively, and do not allow any material to get under the occlusal rests or the guiding planes, if they are present. Seat the partial denture in the mouth, and with magnification, verify that all attachments are fully seated.

Functional method—Apply a tissue-conditioning material such as Lynol* to the relieved tissue surface of the partial denture saddle. Have the patient wear the denture for at least 24

hours, then examine the surface of the impression for completeness and any damage which might have been caused between office visits. Since this method is often employed for distal extensions, check for change in the positional relationship of the saddles to the ridge, which will have resulted in a concurrent change in the relationship of the framework to the teeth. This problem is a potential drawback to the functional impression technique, because a patient can present after wearing the denture for one day with the impression material appearing perfect. However, the material may actually be thinner than it should be due to excessive bruxing or clenching forces over these 24 hours, negating any improvement the relining was meant to achieve.

Step 3

Make a full-arch irreversible hydrocolloid impression with the partial denture in place. As an

*L.D. Caulk Co., Milford, Conn.

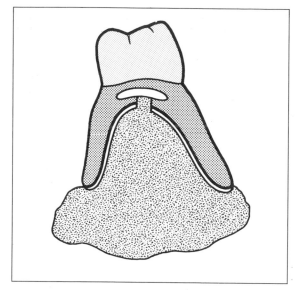

Fig. 8-36 Stone poured into saddle showing small post protruding through hole in acrylic and contacting metal framework.

alternative, the partial denture with its reline impression can be sent to the laboratory without making the overimpression and pouring a cast.

Step 4

In the case of a distal extension removable partial denture, make an opening with about a no. 10 round bur through the impression material and old acrylic until the gingival side of the framework metal casting is exposed. This opening should be made at the most distal aspect of the metal framework. Having done this, when the stone is later poured into the saddle, a small supporting post will protrude from the level of the prevailing tissue surface of the cast and contact the metal of the framework. In this way the framework position will be maintained after removal of the impression material that is supporting the saddle area in proper relation to the rest of the cast (Fig. 8-36).

Step 5

Pour the cast in dental stone. The impression

for this procedure can be handled in one of two ways:

1. Pour the overimpression in stone with the partial denture in place to form a composite cast on which the partial denture is mounted.
2. The impression/denture complex can be presented to the laboratory by itself, in which case the technician first pours stone into the impressions in the saddle(s) and allows it to reach initial set. Then, invert the case onto a patty of wet unset stone. While the cast is roughly the size of a full arch, it does not actually reproduce the teeth. Instead, it supports the partial denture framework during the procedures to follow.

Either technique may be used with equal chance of success. The method for making the reline cast does not really matter. The important question to answer is whether to add the new acrylic by flasking the partial denture, or to add the new acrylic without actually going through the flasking process. Whenever possible, relines should be done on partial dentures without flasking, to eliminate the potential danger of distortion of the partial and significantly reduce errors in vertical dimension resulting from incomplete flask closure. It is generally better practice to use a reline jig and to add one of the dependable, self-curing acrylic resins to the saddle.

Step 6

The procedures outlined below are completed in the laboratory:

1. An occlusal index is made in plaster, and attached to the lower member of a suitable reline jig.
2. The cast is attached to the upper member of the reline jig without removing it from the occlusal index, which at this point is still attached to the lower member.
3. The two halves of the jig are separated at the junction between the occlusal index and

the cast, which at this point still has the partial denture mounted on it.

4. The partial denture is removed from the cast.
5. An appropriate separating medium is applied to the cast and the occlusal index.
6. The surface of the acrylic saddle to be relined with new acrylic is cleaned of all impression material, adhesive, or any debris, and the finish lines are prepared on the old acrylic, as described previously.
7. The partial denture is attached firmly to the plaster occlusal index with sticky wax.
8. The new resin is mixed according to the manufacturer's instructions and carefully placed into the saddles to be relined, so as not to lodge new material under a rest or on guiding planes.
9. The upper half of the jig is now mounted onto the lower half and the mounting nuts tightened. It is at this point that the advantage of the jig over the flask becomes evident. Since with the jig there are no opposing surfaces of plaster for the flash of acrylic to extend between, there is no reason for the two halves of the jig not to seal perfectly together. The flash, in this case, is free to extrude laterally without interfering with closure.
10. The partial denture is processed and finished in the usual manner. Again we see another advantage of the jig over the flask method: since the framework is not imbedded in solid plaster, there is much less danger in disassembling it.

Step 7

Insert the partial denture as with any new partial denture, and check the occlusion, flange extensions, and tissue contacts.

Rebasing partial dentures

Rebasing differs from relining in that the entire denture base is replaced, leaving the relation-ship between the denture teeth and the cast framework unaltered. It is generally done for one of the following reasons:

1. Failure of the acrylic base material over time.
2. Poor polymerization of the acrylic in the processing phase of construction.
3. Desire to change the contour of the outer surfaces of the denture flanges for esthetics, comfort, prevention of food collection, or similar reasons.

The clinical procedures before and after the laboratory phase are nearly identical to those for a reline. The only difference is that the dentist must decide which procedure is needed on the basis of the condition of the acrylic base, and the condition and occlusion of the denture teeth.

Method

Step 1

Make an impression of the tissue-bearing surfaces of the partial denture following the same technique and using the same materials as for a reline. Use the partial denture as a custom tray after creating the necessary internal relief. The primary difference is that the place where the relief ends at the periphery is not as critical in this procedure, since there will be no junction between old and new acrylic materials. Send the impression to the laboratory or pour it in the office with either the partial denture alone or imbedded in an alginate overimpression. If the flanges do not end in a well extended periphery, this can be corrected by border-molding the old denture base prior to making a rebase impression.

Step 2

Make an opening with about a no. 10 round bur through the impression material and old acrylic until the gingival side of the framework metal casting is exposed. This opening should be made at the most distal aspect of the metal framework. When the stone is later poured into the saddle a small supporting post will protrude from the level of the prevailing tissue surface of the cast and contact the metal of the framework. In this manner the position of the framework will be maintained after removal of the impression material which presently supports the saddle area in proper relation to the rest of the cast (Fig. 8-36).

Step 3

Pour the cast in dental stone. Handle the impression for this procedure in one of two ways:

1. Pour the overimpression in stone with the partial denture in place to form a composite cast on which the partial denture is mounted.
2. Present the impression/denture complex to the laboratory by itself, in which case, stone is poured into the impressions in the saddles and allowed to reach initial set. Then, invert the case onto a patty of wet unset stone. While the cast is roughly the size of a full-arch, it does not actually reproduce the teeth, but supports the partial denture framework during the following procedures.

Step 4

The laboratory completes the procedures outlined below:

1. The cast is prepared for mounting on the articulator, including indexing the base. Note that the primary difference between the laboratory procedure for a reline and a rebase is that in a rebase the jig is not used and the partial denture is flasked for processing.
2. The cast is mounted on the mandibular member of an articulator.
3. Using a blockout material, the occlusal surfaces of the denture teeth are isolated in preparation for making a plaster occlusal index, which is attached to the maxillary member of the articulator.
4. The partial denture is removed from the stone cast on the mandibular member of the articulator.
5. The denture teeth are removed from the partial denture by carefully cutting around them with an appropriate bur, being sure to make the cuts at the expense of the base material rather than the teeth.
6. The denture teeth are mounted onto the occlusal index and held in proper position with sticky wax.
7. The remainder of the old acrylic base material is burned off of the framework or otherwise removed.
8. The stability of the positioning of the bare metal framework on the stone cast should be carefully evaluated. The laboratory technician should check carefully the contact between the partial denture framework and the previously developed stone stop at the posterior end of any distal extension. Relying on a "tissue stop" waxed into the framework that was originally made many years before is questionable, since it will sometimes be found that this stop was located on the alveolar ridge area, not on the retromolar pad or other permanent anatomic landmark. Eventually this stop may not be an accurate guidepost for positioning the denture framework. This is much more critical in rebasing than in relining. In relining a fixed jig is used, which maintains the relationship of the framework more accurately since the teeth, when seated into the occlusal index, are still attached to the base material. In rebasing, the framework has lost that relationship and is free to "float" between the tissue surface of the stone cast and the gingival side of the teeth mounted in the occlusal index.
9. The new denture flanges are waxed. The denture teeth are transferred to the new waxup from the occlusal index on the maxillary member of the articulator where they have been temporarily stored in correct position. This is done very simply by closing the articulator into softened baseplate wax which has been built up on the saddle areas

of the framework on the stone cast, which is mounted to the mandibular member of the articulator. Note that it is at this point that one of the indications for doing a rebase rather than a reline is quite obvious. There is total freedom at this step to contour the external surfaces of the flanges of the denture to a more ideal form than was present in the original denture. This advantage does not exist with a reline where the flanges are left as is.

10. The case is now flasked, processed, and finished as with any brand new partial denture.

Step 5

The partial denture is inserted as with any new partial denture. The dentist should check the occlusion, flange extensions, and tissue contact following normal practice for insertion of a new restoration.

References

1. McCracken, W.L. Partial Denture Construction. St. Louis: The C.V. Mosby Co., 1960.
2. McArthur, D.R. Metal posterior teeth for the chronic bruxing patient. J. Prosthet. Dent. 39:578–581, 1978.
3. Schneider, R.L. Custom metal occlusal surfaces for acrylic resin denture teeth. J. Prosthet. Dent. 46:98–101, 1981.
4. Stankewitz, C.G., et al. Adjustment of cast clasps for direct retention. J. Prosthet. Dent. 45:344, 1981.
5. Pirto, M., et al. Enamel bonding plastic materials in modifying the form of abutment teeth for better functioning of partial prosthesis. J. Oral Rehab. 4:1–8, 1977.
6. Jenkins, C.B.G., and Berry, D.C. Modifications of tooth contour by acid etch retained resins for prosthetic purposes. Br. Dent. J. 141:89–90, 1976.
7. Brudvik, J.S., and Nicholls, J.I. Soldering of removable partial dentures. J. Prosthet. Dent. 49:762–765, 1983.
8. Lu, D.P. Chairside replacement of a fractured clasp for removable partial denture. J. Prosthet. Dent. 49:282–285, 1983.
9. Smith, R.A. Clasp repair for removable partial dentures. J. Prosthet. Dent. 29:231, 1973.
10. Smith, R.A., and Rymarz, F.P. Cast clasp transitional removable partial dentures. J. Prosthet. Dent. 22:381, 1969.
11. McCracken, W.L. Partial Denture Construction. St. Louis: The C.V. Mosby Co., 1960, p. 494.
12. Rudd, K.D., et al. Dental Laboratory Procedures. Vol. 3. St. Louis: The C.V. Mosby Co., 1981, p. 441.
13. MacEntee, M.I., et al. The tensile and shear strength of a base metal weld joint used in dentistry. J. Dent. Res. 60:154, 1981.
14. Payne, S.H. A transitional denture. J. Prosthet. Dent. 14:221, 1964.
15. Bailey, L.R. Denture repairs. Chapter 24. *In* S. Winkler (ed.) Essentials of Complete Denture Prosthodontics. Philadelphia: W.B. Saunders Co., 1979.
16. Abbott, F.B., and Wongthai, P. Converting a removable partial denture to a complete interim denture. J. Prosthet. Dent. 49:852–855, 1983.
17. Grady, R.D. Objective criteria for relining distal-extension removable partial dentures: A preliminary report. J. Prosthet. Dent. 49:178–181, 1983.
18. Blatterfein, L. Rebasing procedures for removable partial dentures. J. Prosthet. Dent. 8:441, 1958.
19. Fowler, J.A., et al. Laboratory procedures for the maintenance of a removable partial overdenture. J. Prosthet. Dent. 50:121–126, 1983.
20. Steffel, V.L. Relining removable partial dentures for fit and function. J. Prosthet. Dent. 4:496, 1954.

Additional reading

Abere, D.J. Post-placement care of complete and removable partial dentures. D. Clin. N. Am. 23:143–151, 1979.
Berg, T. I-Bar: Myth and countermyth. D. Clin. N. Am. 23:65–75, 1979.
Berge, M. Bending strength of intact and repaired denture base resins. Acta Odontol. Scand. 41:187–191.
Broering, L.F., and Gooch, W.M. Technique for the repair of removable partial denture backings. J. Prosthet. Dent. 50:582–583, 1983.
Calomeni, A.A. Gold crown fabrication for complete dentures. J. Prosthet. Dent. 50:439–440, 1983.
Frank, R.P., et al. A comparison of the flexibility of wrought wire and cast circumferential clasps. J. Prosthet. Dent. 49:471–476, 1983.
Gaster, B.D., et al. Relining removable partial dentures: Special emphasis on mandibular bilateral distal extension removable partial dentures. R. I. Dent. J. 16:6, 8–9, 12, 1983.
Goska, J.R., et al. A simple, accurate, and quick method of fabricating metal occlusal surfaces for removable partial dentures. Quint. Dent. Technol. 7:405–406, 1983.
Heintz, W.D. Treatment planning and design: Prevention of errors of omission and commission. D. Clin. N. Am. 23:3–12, 1979.
Jochen, D.G., and Caputo, A.A. Composite resin repair of

porcelain denture teeth. J. Prosthet. Dent. 38:673–679, 1977.

Kazanoglu, A., and Smith, E.H. Replacement technique for a broken occlusal rest. J. Prosthet. Dent. 48:621–623, 1982.

Leupold, R.J., and Kratochvil, F.J. An altered-cast procedure to improve tissue support for removable partial dentures. J. Prosthet. Dent. 15:672, 1965.

Lewis, A.J. Failure of removable partial denture castings during service. J. Prosthet. Dent. 39:147–149, 1978.

McCartney, J.W. Occlusal reconstruction and rebase procedure for distal extension removable partial dentures. J. Prosthet. Dent. 43:695–698, 1980.

McCracken, W.L. Partial Denture Construction. St. Louis: The C.V. Mosby Co., 1960.

Powers, W.J., and Connelly, M.E. The immediate replacement of a partial denture abutment tooth. Gen. Dent. 30:234–235, 1982.

Preston, J.D. Preventing ceramic failures when integrating fixed and removable prostheses. D. Clin. N. Am. 23:37–52, 1979.

Reitz. P.V., and Weiner, M.G. Fabrication of interim acrylic resin removable dentures with clasps. J. Prosthet. Dent. 40:686–688, 1978.

Rudd, K.D., et al. Relining and rebasing. Chapter 14. Dental Laboratory Procedures. Vol. 3. St. Louis: The C.V. Mosby Co., 1981.

Shay, J.S., and Mattingly, S.L. Technique for the immediate repair of removable partial denture facings. J. Prosthet. Dent. 47:104–106, 1982.

Chapter 9

Adjunct Procedures

This chapter presents detailed methods for adjunct procedures referred to elsewhere in the text. In addition to their usefulness in treatments for modifying and preserving existing dental restorations, the following procedures are also used in routine patient treatment.

The stereomicroscope

The intricate procedures of prosthodontics involve the smallest of objects, and fits that must be as near to perfect as possible. Precise detail is often not clearly visible to the naked eye. Unquestionably, the stereomicroscope is one of the best aids in accomplishing high quality prosthodontic treatment.

The primary value of the stereomicroscope is in indirect procedures where an object is examined in the laboratory or at chairside.[1] Stereomagnification is rarely used for procedures directly in the mouth of the patient, either with actual microscopes in the $10 \times$ to $20 \times$ range, or with the more familiar "loops" that are usually in the $2 \times$ to $4 \times$ range.

Stereomagnification can be used for the following:

1. Impression evaluation
2. Cast and die examination
3. Surveying dies for undercuts
4. Die trimming
5. Waxing margins
6. Attaching sprues to wax patterns
7. Evaluating castings
8. Evaluating fit of casting on die
9. Margin finishing and polishing
10. Fit of castings on the tooth preparation
11. Rotary instrument evaluation
12. Hand instrument sharpening

The authors recommend the Model 42 stereomicroscope by the American Optical Company.* It is ideal for the above uses because it has a variable turret type adjustment for $10 \times$ to $20 \times$ magnification, adequate workspace for both hands, and a completely enclosed gear mechanism such that grindings will not interfere with the movement of the worm gear. Use it with a good concentrated light source such as the Sunnex Model 703,** which is equipped with a gooseneck for easy adjustment and provides an illumination of 1,000 candlepower at 12 inches. A 12-volt halogen bulb will provide ample light while giving off an acceptable amount of heat. Some practitioners and technicians find a two-lamp setup more versatile.

Impression evaluation

Every impression should be examined under the stereomicroscope immediately after re-

---

*American Optical Corp., Buffalo, N.Y.
**Sunnex, Needham, Mass.

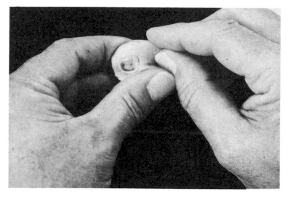

Fig. 9-1a Impression viewed with the naked eye.

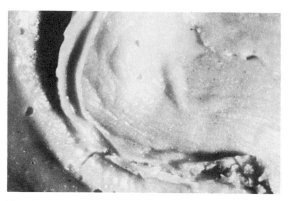

Fig. 9-1b Impression viewed under the stereomicroscope.

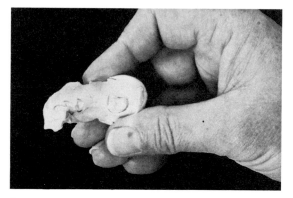

Fig. 9-2a Untrimmed stone cast viewed with the naked eye.

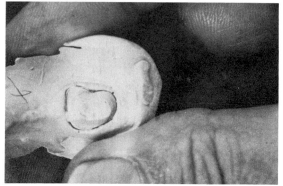

Fig. 9-2b Untrimmed stone cast viewed with the stereomicroscope.

moval from the mouth. Almost every possible defect in the impression can be seen with great reliability under the microscope (Figs. 9-1a and b). Do not wait until the cast has been poured and separated to decide that a finish line is missing. At that point, the patient must be recalled, the temporary removed, and the tooth reanesthetized, a time-consuming and unnecessary inconvenience.

Cast and die examination

Assuming that the impression was examined when it was made, it is essential to verify the absence of bubbles in the stone mix and pouring. Occasionally, an unusable finish line will be detected here, although it may have appeared perfect when the impression was examined. As with the impression, the untrimmed cast can be evaluated more accurately under the stereomicroscope than with the naked eye (Figs. 9-2a and b).

Surveying dies

Surveying dies can be particularly helpful when constructing a crown under an existing partial denture or when improving retention for a clasp. In either case, the cast or die can be examined under magnification to evaluate the result of any alterations made to the surface. When making a new crown under an existing partial denture, a slight undercut sometimes occurs at the gingival end of a wall that was being realigned for better guiding plane or clasp design.

Die trimming

One of the best uses for the stereomicroscope is trimming excess stone from below a finish line on a die. A sharp scalpel blade with a pointed tip, a discoid-cleoid, or any similar sharp instrument can be used to a much higher level of precision under $20 \times$ magnification than with the naked eye alone (Fig. 9-3).

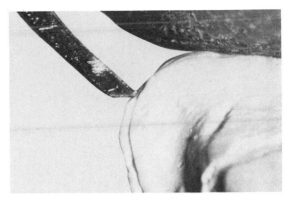

Fig. 9-3 Die trimming under the stereomicroscope.

Margin waxing

Most likely the highest-priority use for the stereomicroscope is waxing margins. Laboratory technicians accustomed to waxing all margins under the stereomicroscope will do so exclusively. One of the many advantages is that the margins on the stone die undergo less abrasion. The clear, close-up view helps the technician avoid carving into the stone accidentally, and because the margin is carved properly the first time, the number of passes with the instrument is substantially reduced (Fig. 9-4).

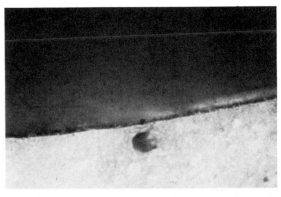

Fig. 9-4 Wax margin as seen using the stereomicroscope showing not only the fine precision possible in carving, but also the fact that a potentially troublesome bubble in the stone is not on the finish line.

Casting evaluation and fit on die

Significant treatment time can be saved by examining the inside of the casting prior to taking the casting to the mouth, and by checking the completeness of seating on the die. Improving the final fit of the casting is also important. Using a stereomicroscope for this purpose, one realizes that numerous small blebs inside a casting cannot be seen with the naked eye. These defects often appear in and around the cusp tips and are caused by small amounts of air entrapped during investing. Upon removal of the positive defects with the aid of the stereomicroscope, observe that the area of adjustment is confined to a much smaller area than if the work is done without magnification. A casting can be forced onto the die yet not seat on the tooth,

because a small bleb will dig into the die, but not the dentin. Also, the integrity of the marginal fit is best appreciated with magnification.

Another valuable application of the stereomicroscope during fitting of the casting to the stone die is the use of a machinist's marking dye.* This material is painted on the stone die or over a die spacer, if one was used, before trying the casting on the die. When the casting is then tried on the painted die, any area that prevents complete seating is marked on the inside of the casting. By carefully adjusting the marked areas

*Layout fluid, Dayton Rogers Manufacturing Co., Minneapolis, Minn.

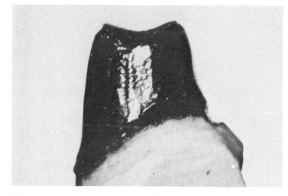

Fig. 9-5a Stone die painted with machinist's marking dye.

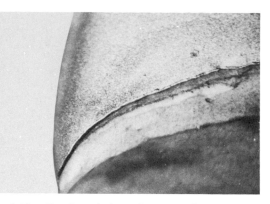

Fig. 9-5b Casting tried on die, not well seated because of interference on the inner surface.

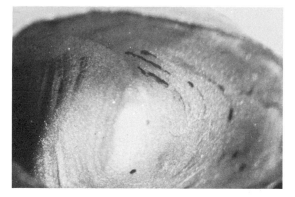

Fig. 9-5c Red pencil marks on inner surface of casting.

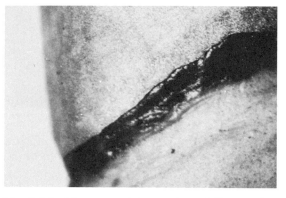

Fig. 9-5d More complete seating of the casting after removal of interferences.

and then repeating this step, complete seating on the die can be attained without abrading the die or losing retention, which can occur from indiscriminate grinding inside the casting. This material is better than more traditional ones because the same spot will tend to mark more often before it is necessary to paint on another layer of the marking dye (Figs. 9-5a to d).

Clinical evaluation of casting fit on tooth preparation

The final step to take with the stereomicroscope to improve prosthodontic treatment is to use marking or indicator material to show high spots that keep the casting from seating perfectly on the tooth. Here, use a silicone wash by placing a mix of injection viscosity silicone material inside the crown, then place the crown on the tooth. After setting, remove the crown with the wash material inside, and examine under the stereomicroscope. The interference areas show up as perforations through the material to the gold.

Mark the perforation through the silicone wash material with a pencil, and remove the wash material (Figs. 9-6a and b). The "high spots" are now marked on the inside surface of the casting and are easily identifiable under the stereomicroscope (Fig. 9-6c).

Another alternative is the more traditional mixture of gold rouge and chloroform. Several newer materials are also presently on the market for this purpose. The gold rouge and chloro-

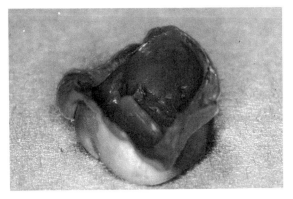

Fig. 9-6a Silicone wash inside crown indicating interferences when crown is tried on tooth.

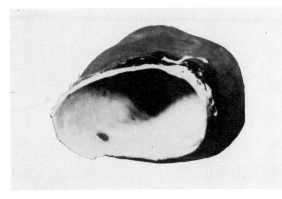

Fig. 9-6b A different silicone wash with red pencil mark through perforation of wash material.

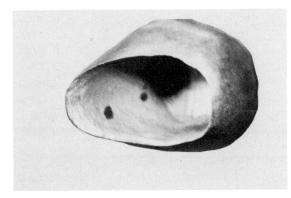

Fig. 9-6c Resulting red pencil marks after removal of silicone wash material.

form alternative is particularly useful when adjusting a partial denture framework to a new crown.

Check-Bite impression technique

Full-arch casts are mounted either with occlusal registrations of some type, or by hand, if the occlusion is stable enough. This is recommended for multiple restorations, partial dentures, and bridges. However, for some single-unit restorations the Check-Bite* technique is ideal.

The following are some of the advantages of the Check-Bite technique over full-arch casts or individual quadrant casts:

1. Both maxillary and mandibular impressions are made simultaneously.
2. The occlusal relationship, if the technique is performed correctly, is likely to be better than those achieved with methods that use an interocclusal record.
3. There is a saving of materials, and the case can be mounted on a small-quadrant articulator rather than a full-mouth one, although this is not as important as the previous two advantages.

The Check-Bite impression technique is particularly adaptable to procedures involving Class I inlays, in that there is no need to generate a separate trimmed die in order to contend with gingival finish lines, since all the finish lines are quite accessible on the occlusal surface of the quadrant cast.

The method described here uses hydrocolloid impression material (reversible alginate), as the tray's design dictates. Polysulfide rubber material should not be used because of its sensitivity to excessive and uneven thicknesses. However, some of the newer polyvinylsiloxanes, which do not have the thickness problems of the older elastomers, can be used, but the authors prefer the hydrocolloid material for Check-Bite impressions.

*Coe Laboratories, Inc., Chicago, Ill.

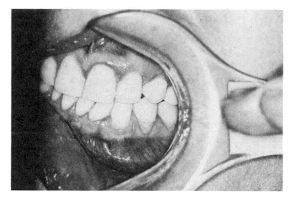

Fig. 9-7 Occlusion on opposite side of arch checked for perfect closure.

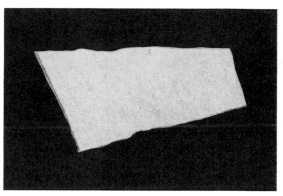

Fig. 9-8 Paper used with Check-Bite tray.

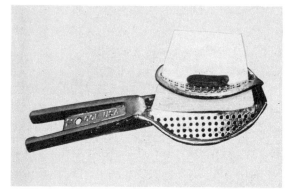

Fig. 9-9 Tray ready for filling with reversible alginate, showing soft periphery wax holding paper in position.

Method

Step 1

Try the tray in the patient's mouth to verify two conditions: *(1)* that the bar connecting the two halves of the tray will pass distally to the last tooth in the arch, clearing the tissue, and allowing the patient to close the teeth fully into occlusion; and *(2)* that the two halves of the tray are far enough apart to accommodate the arches when the patient closes. These trays can easily be bent accidentally—if this is the case, the tray must be carefully bent back open. Check arch accommodation by having the patient close fully

into CO and verify complete closure by examining the relationship of the teeth on the opposite side of the mouth (Fig. 9-7). This relationship must be the same when the tray is in the mouth as it is when the tray is not present.

Step 2

Place a special paper separator into the slots in each half of the tray to form a barrier between the material making the maxillary impression and that making the mandibular impression. This paper is 0.001 inches thick when dry, but compresses to nearly zero when wet, as during occlusal loading in the impression procedure (Fig. 9-8). A small amount of soft red periphery wax on each side of the tray where the paper exits the slot will hold it in place (Fig. 9-9).

Step 3

Load the hydrocolloid into the sides of the tray from a tube, and ensure that the material is viscous enough to hold its position. A 4-by-4-inch gauze wrapped around the loaded tray will prevent the material from slumping while it is placed into the tempering bath of the conditioner. The material is tempered according to manufacturer instructions.

Step 4

Dry the field, inject the preparation with hydro-

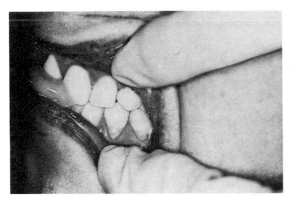

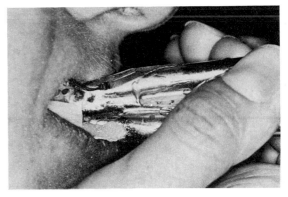

Fig. 9-10 Occlusion on the opposite side checked again for complete closure after seating of Check-Bite tray.

Fig. 9-11 Patient supporting tray during cooling.

colloid material from a syringe, and place the tray in the mouth such that full closing is possible just as during the initial try-in. The mounting will be correct later on the articulator only if the teeth are in CO at this point. Check the occlusal relationship on the opposite side of the arch again at this time to be certain that the proper relationship is maintained (Fig. 9-10).

Step 5

Leave the tray in place for 5 minutes and run cold water through the tubing of the tray. During this time, the patient or the assistant supports the tubes so that they will not be a downward force and cause distortion of the impression (Fig. 9-11). Water should be run through the tray by suction rather than by pressure. Place one of the tubes in an open container of water and apply a vacuum to the other one from the dental unit. Hand-soldered joints make these trays extremely vulnerable to cracking and leaks, and "pulling" instead of "pushing" the water through under pressure will prevent a small opening from causing a flood of water into the patient's mouth. After the hydrocolloid has set, remove the tray after instructing the patient to open with a quick movement.

Step 6

Pour the impression in the following manner,

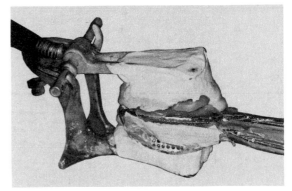

Fig. 9-12 Check-Bite tray with impression poured on both sides, mounted in quadrant articulator prior to removing resulting quadrant casts from the impression.

which is the most expeditious regimen and which does not compromise accuracy:

1. Pour the opposing side of the impression first, using a mixture of yellow stone and either slurry water or a small amount of fast-setting impression plaster to hasten the set.
2. When this is set—usually within a few minutes—pour the side with the impression of the preparation in a densite die stone such as Vel Mix.
3. When the second pour has set, mount the two casts, *without separating them from the impression,* in a quadrant articulator (Fig. 9-12).

4. After the mounting plaster has set, open the articulator and remove the impression from the cast on which it remained.

5. Close the aritculator and verify that the casts are in perfect relationship. If the dentist was careful to be sure the patient was in perfect occlusion by observing the occlusal relationship of the opposite teeth as soon as the tray was placed, there is little chance for error.

Step 7

If the casts will not be mounted within 1 or 2 hours after pouring, take the following precaution. When the second cast is poured, be sure that some stone contacts the stone at the anterior and posterior ends of the hardened first cast. Any distortion of the hydrocolloid caused by water loss over a prolonged period of time cannot change the relationship of the two casts, since they are temporarily connected together at the ends. These attachments can be broken apart easily after mounting.

Indirect temporary restorations

The indirect acrylic temporary technique is the best all-around method for constructing an interim restoration during fabrication of fixed restorations, providing several advantages over preformed crowns and direct acrylic restorations.[2-3] Not the least of these advantages is the potential for achieving a significantly higher quality temporary restoration in terms of marginal fit and surface integrity of the acrylic, which promotes better tissue health (Fig. 9-13).

Method

The method is particularly significant when used with restorations of teeth under existing partial dentures, because it generates an acrylic temporary restoration that duplicates the tooth contour or crown as it currently exists. This means the clinical crown must be a relatively

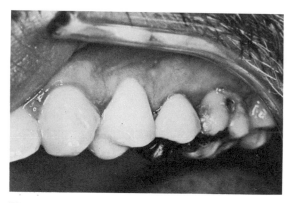

Fig. 9-13 Temporary crown, made indirectly on the maxillary left first premolar, showing excellent tissue response after two weeks.

complete form. If it is not, as with a fractured cusp or a broken facing on a crown, there will be enough form present to arrive at nearly all the needed contour. Often the missing form can be temporarily reconstructed in the mouth with a soft wax, an overimpression made over the wax, and the wax removed. Better yet, the missing form can be developed on a diagnostic waxup, and the cast duplicated for use in this as well as other procedures.

Only by this method can a temporary restoration be quickly and reliably generated which will allow the patient to wear the partial denture while the new crown is being constructed. Proceed as follows:

Step 1

Make a form of the outer contour of the teeth in the involved area, either from the diagnostic cast or the mouth, if the complete required contour is present. Make the form with an overimpression of irreversible hydrocolloid, or by thermoforming a sheet of polypropyline plastic over a stone duplicate of the diagnostic waxup cast (Fig. 9-14). When making a simple single crown, include only the particular quadrant in which the crown is located. *If, however, the case involves a crown under an existing partial denture, it is essential to include the entire arch in both the overimpression and the impression of*

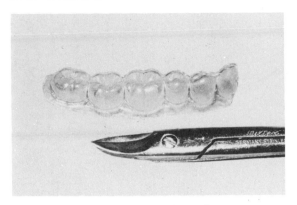

Fig. 9-14   Clear plastic form trimmed.

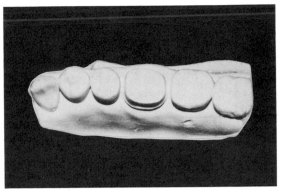

Fig. 9-15   Fast-setting plaster cast of quadrant in which preparation was done.

the preparation. This is because the added stability and indexing potential of a full-arch cast into a full-arch overimpression will make the temporary crown an accurate duplication of the original tooth and thus allow the partial denture to seat on it.

Step 2

Store the irreversible hydrocolloid overimpression form in a humidor or set aside the plastic form. The form will be used after completion of the preparation in the mouth. Prepare the tooth as usual, satisfying all requirements of the situation at hand. With a crown preparation under an existing partial denture, try in the partial denture during preparation to verify that there is adequate reduction for such features of the framework as the occlusal rest, guide plane, or retentive clasp, whichever are present.

Step 3

After completing the preparation, make an irreversible hydrocolloid impression, involving the same area as the overimpression. Again, it is essential that when a crown under an existing partial denture is being made, a full-arch impression of the preparation is made. Pour the impression of the preparation in a fast-setting plaster, but do not pour in dental or densite

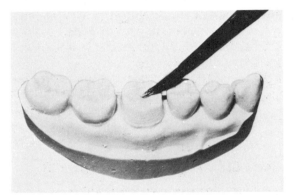

Fig. 9-16   Preparation on cast being lubricated.

stone because: *(1)* the material must set quickly, and *(2)* it needs to be easily broken out of the cured acrylic temporary without damaging the temporary. After it has set, separate the cast from the impression and trim it so that it will fit completely into the overimpression or plastic form (Fig. 9-15). Lubricate the tooth preparation on the plaster cast with a tin-foil substitute (Fig. 9-16).

Step 4

Select the appropriate shade of self-curing acrylic resin, and mix in a dappen dish to a consistency of heavy cream, which will readily

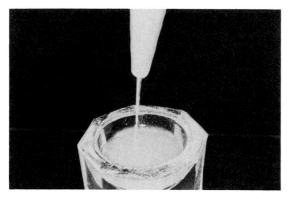

Fig. 9-17 Acrylic powder is added to liquid to make a runny mix.

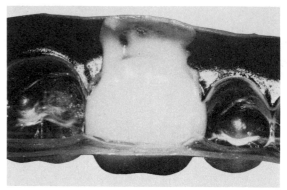

Fig. 9-18 Acrylic flowed into appropriate tooth of clear plastic form.

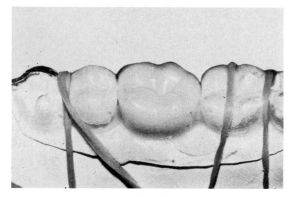

Fig. 9-19 Assembly of clear plastic form, wet acrylic, and plaster cast.

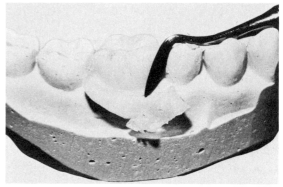

Fig. 9-20 Chipping away gross excess.

flow, adding the powder into the monomer (Fig. 9-17). Place into the area of the prepared tooth in the overimpression or plastic form (Fig. 9-18). The amount to use will be learned with some practice, but the important point to remember is to avoid using an excessive amount. Any excess will tend to extrude over the occlusal surfaces of the adjacent teeth between the plaster cast and the form and prevent the cast from seating all the way into the form. If this occurs, the occlusion on the temporary restoration will be high when tried in the mouth. Also, with a crown under an existing partial denture, there will be less chance for perfect seating of the partial denture because all of the contours of the temporary will be elevated.

Step 5

Place the plaster cast all the way into the form and wrap a rubberband around the assembly (Fig. 9-19). Put the assembly into a heated water bath and allow the acrylic to cure for about 10 minutes. Remove from the water bath and separate the plaster cast from the form. The temporary restoration will usually stay on the cast. If it does not, place it on the cast.

Step 6

Verify that the temporary restoration is complete, add to any deficient area and place the temporary, still on the plaster cast, back in the

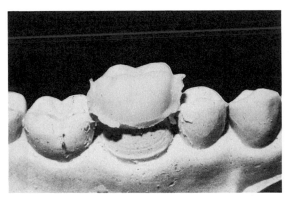

Fig. 9-21a Set acrylic crown removed from plaster cast.

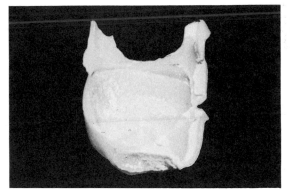

Fig. 9-21b Resulting acrylic crown with minimal excess.

heated water bath for a few minutes to cure any added acrylic. For crowns under an existing partial denture, avoid adding excessive contour anywhere that might later interfere with seating of the partial denture. Chip away gross excess around the gingival margins (Fig. 9-20). Remove the temporary from the plaster cast (Figs. 9-21a and b).

Step 7

Finish with acrylic trimming stones and/or burs (Fig. 9-22). The margin areas should be finished under the microscope. The greatest advantages of this method over preformed temporaries is a better margin fit and contour for tissue health. But without proper final margin finishing, this benefit will be lost.

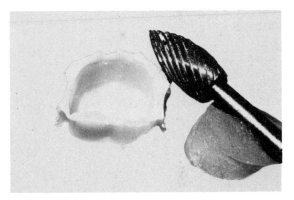

Fig. 9-22 Typical positioning of acrylic trimming bur.

Step 8

Try in the temporary restoration, adjust the occlusion and polish the restoration (Figs. 9-23a to c). It is then cemented with an appropriate temporary cement. In the case of a crown under an existing partial denture, try in the denture with the crown in place prior to cementation to be certain that it fits properly. Make any necessary adjustments in the acrylic so that the partial denture seats completely prior to cementing the temporary.

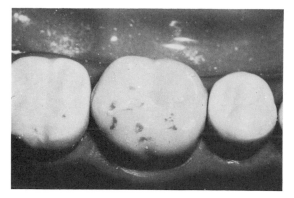

Fig. 9-23a Temporary acrylic crown with occlusion marked.

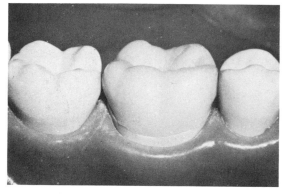

Fig. 9-23b Temporary acrylic crown in place.

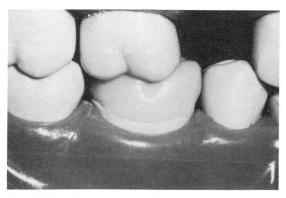

Fig. 9-23c Temporary acrylic crown in occlusion.

Pindex system

Many different methods have been used to develop the removable dies used in constructing fixed prosthodontic restorations. One of the most useful and reliable is the Pindex system.* The essential features of this system are:

1. Perfectly parallel holes drilled into the cast by a special drill press.
2. Precision brass dowel pins that can be cemented into the holes to result in all pins being parallel.
3. Plastic sleeves that fit over the brass pins, and form plastic linings in the base after the base is poured. In this way the pins do not seat into stone, but into the plastic sleeves.
4. Stability of removable dies.

The Pindex system uses several different types of pins. Both long and short brass pins, along with their respective white and grey plastic sleeves, are most often used (Figs. 9-24a and b). The grey sleeves have flat flanges which, after pouring of the base, aid in placing the die without gouging the stone. Both the white and the grey sleeves are designed to allow ease of placement in tight spaces, such as where the pins end up very close together because of tooth size. The Dual-Pin, a variation of the Pindex system by the same manufacturer, is particularly useful in very narrow teeth, like the mandibular anteriors.

The other major piece of equipment needed is the "drill." This consists of a 3450 rpm motor which drives a chuck-mounted twist drill residing below a worktable with a center hole (Fig. 9-25). When the stone cast is placed on the work table, the entire motor assembly with its rotating twist drill is raised to a prescribed height, creating a hole in the cast to later receive the pin. The final critical feature of the drill is a light that shines down on the cast directly in line with the twist drill, allowing a fine degree of accuracy in placing the holes, which would oth-

*Whaledent International, New York, N.Y.

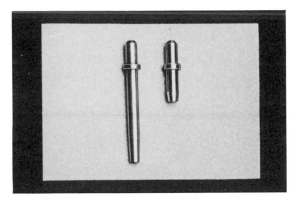

Fig. 9-24a Pindex pins, long and short.

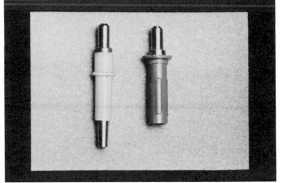

Fig. 9-24b Sleeves on appropriate pins.

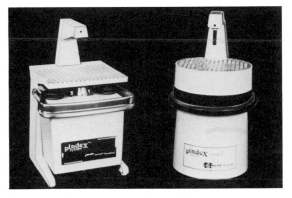

Fig. 9-25 Two versions of the drill.

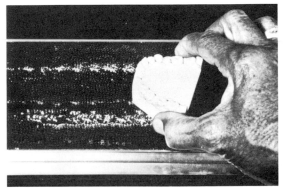

Fig. 9-26 Smoothing the base of the cast prior to drilling holes.

erwise be difficult to obtain because the drill is operating from below the cast, out of sight. The steps creating a cast with removable dies follow.[4]

Step 1

Pour the full-arch impression in either a standard densite die stone or epoxy. At least 15 mm of stone must be left between the occlusal surfaces and the base of the cast. After the stone has set, trim the base on a cast trimmer, assuring that it is generally perpendicular to the occlusal plane. In cases involving very unusual or abnormal tooth inclination this requirement may need to be varied. The variations are beyond the scope of this book, but suffice it to say that experience will soon make the operator wary of this particular problem in relation to the angle of pin placement.

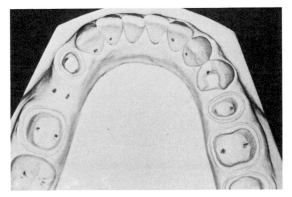

Fig. 9-27 Holes to be drilled in base plotted on occlusal surfaces with a felt-tipped pen.

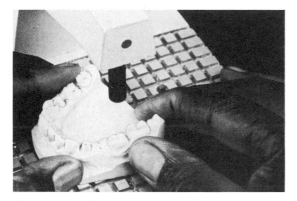

Fig. 9-28 Drilling operation using light beam to locate cast so that each hole drilled on the underside of the base is in line with a previously plotted point on the occlusal surface.

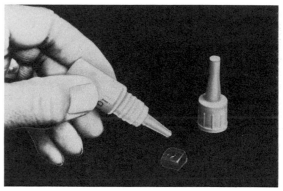

Fig. 9-29 Cyanoacrylate cement being placed into a wax form.

Step 2

Smooth the base of the cast on a flat surface covered with sandpaper. Ensure that the cast is perfectly flat prior to drilling the holes (Fig. 9-26). Using a small, sharp, felt-tipped pen, plot the position of each pin on the occlusal surfaces of the teeth (Fig. 9-27). The primary requirements here are: *(1)* a certain minimum distance must be left between pins, *(2)* two pinholes are placed in each prepared tooth, and *(3)* an adequate number (usually two) pinholes are placed in each section that will be removable, even though it has no preparations. It is important to understand that once the base has been poured and the cast divided into sections with or without preparations, each one of the parts needs its own pins for retention into the base.

Step 3

Let the cast dry thoroughly, usually for 24 hours, for proper operation of the drill. Place the cast, base down, on the worktable and start the motor. Align the holes one at a time under the light pointer, and raise the motor and twist drill assembly to drill the holes. Raise the twist drill all the way to the built-in stop of the unit to assure that the shoulder, which is a part of the twist drill, will penetrate the stone to the proper depth for complete seating of the pin (Fig. 9-28).

Step 4

Air-blow the shavings from the holes, and prepare to cement the pins by making a small wax form and placing a small amount of cyanoacrylate cement in it (Fig. 9-29). Avoid contacting the skin with this cement. Discard the small wax form afterwards, to protect other people from accidental exposure.

Step 5

Take a short pin by its longer end in a pair of pliers which will hold the pin securely. With the other hand, pick up a small bead of the cement on a small instrument such as a Thomas no. 2 wax applicator, and place it in the opening of the hole toward the center of the stone cast. Immediately place the pin into the hole. This type of cement acts by chelating the stone and the reaction starts immediately, so work very quickly, or the stone will start to soften and prevent the pin from properly seating.

Step 6

Seat the rest of the short pins in holes toward the center, seating the long pins in the holes toward the outside of the cast. Clean off any excess cement before attempting to seat the sleeves (Fig. 9-30). Place a thin coat of tin-foil

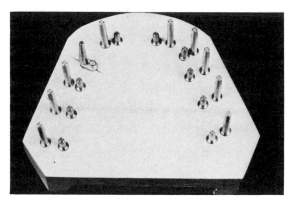

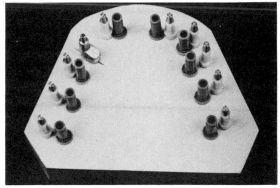

Fig. 9-30 All short and long Pindex pins in place. Note the different type of pin in the mandibular right first premolar position. This variation is called a *Dual-Pin*, and is used in very tight quarters.

Fig. 9-31 White and grey plastic sleeves positioned over appropriate pins.

substitute or other separating medium on the base of the cast and allow to dry.

Step 7

Seat a grey sleeve over each short pin, orienting it so the flange touches the cast, and the flat edge of the flange is facing the long pin. Place a white sleeve over each long pin, and observe that this leaves a portion of the longer end of the long pin exposed. The reason for this will become obvious when the base is poured (Fig. 9-31).

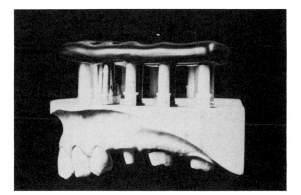

Fig. 9-32 Red carding wax covering ends of pins.

Step 8

Position a strip of carding wax or soft periphery wax on the ends of the long pins so that it also covers the end of the grey sleeves on the short pins (Fig. 9-32).

Step 9

Pour the base. The base form designed for use for the Pindex system can also be used in developing a split-cast mounting. This base form is filled with stone and the cast is placed into the stone with the pins down until they rest on the bottom of the form. The base can also be easily and conveniently poured by simply vibrat-ing some stone around the pin sleeves and onto the base of the cast, and then inverting the cast onto a patty of stone. The authors recommend wrapping the cast in standard duct tape before pouring the base. This is quick and has one great advantage over the previous two methods in that a tight seal is formed all around, which will keep stone from seeping down the sides of the cast and onto the preparations. Remove the cast from the base after the new stone hardens (Fig. 9-33).

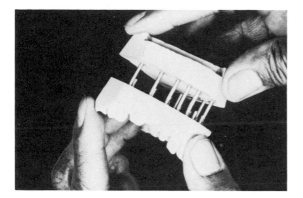

Fig. 9-33 Cast being removed from base.

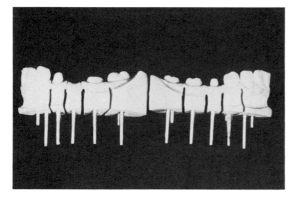

Fig. 9-34a Saw cuts made in cast from gingival aspect, thus obviating bringing the saw blade too close to the finish lines.

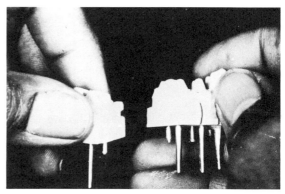

Fig. 9-34b Breaking the cast.

Step 10

Section the cast into individual dies such that the cuts are parallel to the pins and the finish lines of the preparations are protected during the process. The simplest way to section is as follows:

1. Cut out the stone representing the palate if it is present.
2. Replace the cast on the base.
3. Cut between each preparation and the adjacent section. Sometimes this will mean cutting between two preparations, while at other times you will be cutting between a preparation and a section representing uncut teeth. In any event, the cut should be made from the preparation side of the cast only if the saw blade will fit without endangering the finish lines of the preparations.
4. If the finish line is very close to the adjacent tooth, then cut from the underside of the cast after removing it from the base. In this manner, a small amount of stone can be left uncut just adjacent to the preparation finish line, protecting this critical area. Apply a slight force to break this uncut stone, eliminating the need for placing the saw near the finish line in tight areas (Figs. 9-34a and b).

Step 11

Trim each die to eliminate excess stone below the finish line, always using the stereomicroscope. Mount the case in the articulator. Boil out the wax that was placed over the ends of the

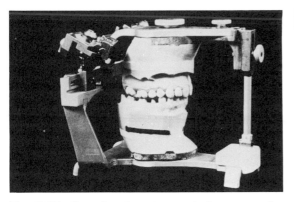

Fig. 9-35 Completed cast mounted on an articulator.

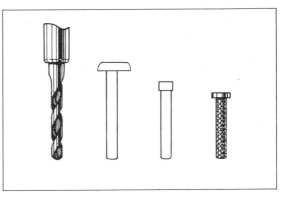

Fig. 9-36 Components of the VIP pin system.

pins and their sleeves, leaving the ends of the long outside pins exposed and available for removing the dies (Fig. 9-35).

VIP pin system

Since nylon bristles were first used for constructing castings that had pins as their integral retentive feature, many different systems and techniques have been advocated. The one presented below is a complete pin system for use in creating castings made of either gold or porcelain-fused-to-metal, which are retained by parallel pins cemented into holes in the dentin.

The VIP (vertical insertion pins) system consists of four parts (Fig. 9-36):

1. A twist drill .024 inches in diameter.
2. Plastic impression pins, .017 inches in diameter, with small heads for retention in the impression material.
3. Iridioplatinum pins for use in the casting itself. These pins are headless, serrated, and approximately .007 inches in diameter. The gold grips the serrations during casting.
4. An aluminum pin for making an acrylic temporary restoration.

The advantage the system has over some others is the calibration, the gradually decreasing sizes of the parts, and the fact that, in contrast to the original nylon bristle, the resulting retentive pin is made of a high-modulus steel and not the same alloy that makes up the casting.

Method

Step 1

Make the preparations as dictated by the particular case. Refer to earlier chapters for the specific details of the various applications. Plot the holes on the preparation according to need for retention at specific points.

Step 2

Drill the holes with the twist drill in the kit in harmony with any other retentive features of the preparation. The holes should be parallel to each other and drilled at least 2 mm into the dentin. Place an impression pin into each hole, and examine for parallelism. Any pinhole out of line must be replaced by one in another location. Avoid this error if possible, and make the impression with the material of choice. Pour the impression in a densite stone.

Step 3

Remove the cast from the impression, and the pins from the cast. Use a twisting motion, but not tipping, to avoid breaking any stone around the pins. After constructing, trimming, and mounting the removable die, lubricate it. Place an iridioplatinum pin from the kit into each hole in the die and begin the waxup by flowing wax to connect all of the pins in a given die. Proceed with the waxup as usual.

Step 4

Make the casting and try it in. The VIP system usually produces minimal complications during try-in. If problems do occur, paint the pins with a mixture of gold rouge and chloroform, and after attempting to insert the casting, examine it again under the stereomicroscope for areas of interference.

If the problem cannot be corrected by slight relief, remake the casting taking particular care to determine if any nonparallel condition exists. Do not cut off or bend any of the pins because they interfere with seating. In the first case, the pin should not have been used if it is not really essential and cutting off a pin would eliminate necessary retention; in the second, stress may be created in the tooth if a pin is bent.

Step 5

Cementation is usually uneventful, except for the fact that it is important to get cement into the holes. This can best be done using a lentulo spiral, or by simply forcing it into the holes with a small instrument. Do not rely on cement placed only on the casting, as this will be wiped up along the pin as the pin enters the hole.

References

1. Oliva, R.A., et al. Use of the stereomicroscope in fixed prosthodontics. J. Dent. Educ. 46:688–671, 1982.
2. Fisher, D.W., et al. Indirect temporary restorations. J. Am. Dent. Assoc. 82:160–163, 1971.
3. Shillingburg, H.T., et al. Preparations for Cast Gold Restorations. Chicago: Quintessence Publ. Co., 1974, pp. 155–167.
4. Pindex Operating Instruction Manual. Whaledent International, New York, N.Y.

Index